GLYCEMIC INDEX FOOD GUIDE CHART FOR SENIORS 2024

Essential Dietary Insights for Managing Diabetes and More

Megan T. Fred

INTRODUCTION

Welcome to the "Glycemic Index Food Guide Chart for Seniors 2024." As we age, maintaining optimal health becomes increasingly important, and one of the key factors in achieving this is understanding how the foods we eat affect our bodies. This guide is designed to provide seniors with the knowledge and tools needed to make informed dietary choices based on the glycemic index (GI) of foods.

The glycemic index is a measure of how quickly a food raises blood glucose levels after consumption. Foods are ranked on a scale from 0 to 100, with higher values indicating a rapid spike in blood sugar. For seniors, managing blood sugar levels is crucial for overall health, as it can help prevent and manage conditions like diabetes, heart disease, and obesity.

How to Use This Guide

This guide is structured to be both informative and practical. It starts with foundational knowledge about the glycemic index, including its definition, measurement, and the differences between glycemic index and glycemic load. The guide then delves into the benefits of low GI foods, especially tailored to the needs of seniors.

We explore the factors that affect the glycemic index of foods, helping you understand why certain foods are classified as high or low GI. You will find comprehensive charts categorizing foods by their glycemic index, making it easy to choose the best options for your diet.

Meal planning and recipes are included to provide practical examples of how to incorporate low GI foods into your daily routine. Additionally, this guide addresses the role of glycemic index in managing chronic conditions, offering valuable insights for those with diabetes, heart disease, or weight management goals.

We also provide shopping tips to help you make the best choices while grocery shopping, and a FAQ section to answer common questions and dispel myths about the glycemic index. Finally, we include a list of resources for further reading and support.

Our Commitment

This guide is not just a book; it is a commitment to empowering seniors with the knowledge needed to make healthier choices. Whether you are looking to manage a chronic condition, improve your overall health, or simply make informed dietary choices, the "Glycemic Index Food Guide Chart for Seniors 2024" is here to support you on your journey.

We hope this guide becomes a valuable resource for you, providing both the information and inspiration needed to live a healthier, more vibrant life.

TABLE OF CONTENTS

Chapter 1: What is Glycemic Index?

1.1 Definition and Explanation

The glycemic index (GI) is a scientific measure that ranks carbohydrate-containing foods according to their effect on blood glucose (sugar) levels. Developed by Dr. David Jenkins and his colleagues in the early 1980s at the University of Toronto, the glycemic index provides a valuable tool for understanding how different foods influence blood sugar.

Definition

The glycemic index assigns a numerical value to foods based on their impact on blood glucose levels over a specified period. This scale ranges from 0 to 100, with pure glucose serving as the reference point with a GI of 100. Foods are categorized as:

- **Low GI (55 or less):** Foods that cause a slow, gradual increase in blood glucose levels.
- **Medium GI (56 to 69):** Foods that cause a moderate increase in blood glucose levels.
- **High GI (70 or above):** Foods that cause a rapid spike in blood glucose levels.

Explanation

The glycemic index measures the rate at which the carbohydrates in a food are digested, absorbed, and converted into glucose in the bloodstream. Here's how it works:

1. **Digestion and Absorption:** When you consume carbohydrates, they are broken down into simpler sugars during digestion. These sugars are then absorbed into the bloodstream, causing blood glucose levels to rise.
2. **Blood Glucose Response:** The speed and extent to which blood glucose levels rise after consuming a food depends on the type of carbohydrate it contains, its

fiber content, and how it is processed and prepared. High GI foods are rapidly digested and absorbed, leading to a quick and significant rise in blood glucose levels. In contrast, low GI foods are digested and absorbed more slowly, resulting in a gradual increase in blood glucose levels.

3. **GI Testing Procedure:** To determine the GI of a food, a group of healthy individuals consumes a portion of the test food containing 50 grams of available carbohydrates. Blood samples are taken at regular intervals over the next two hours to measure the blood glucose response. This response is compared to the response elicited by consuming an equal amount of pure glucose or white bread. The average blood glucose response to the test food is then expressed as a percentage of the response to the reference food, resulting in the food's GI value.

The glycemic index is a crucial concept for anyone looking to maintain a healthy diet and manage blood sugar levels effectively. By choosing low GI foods, individuals, especially seniors, can achieve better health outcomes and improve their quality of life.

1.2 How the Glycemic Index is Measured

The glycemic index (GI) is determined through a standardized testing process that involves measuring the blood glucose response to a specific food. This process helps classify foods based on how they affect blood sugar levels, providing a valuable tool for dietary planning, particularly for individuals managing conditions like diabetes. Here's a detailed explanation of how the glycemic index is measured:

Step-by-Step Process

1. **Selection of Participants**
   - A group of 10 to 12 healthy individuals, typically volunteers, is chosen for the testing.
   - These participants should have normal blood glucose regulation to ensure consistent and reliable results.
2. **Preparation of Test Foods**
   - The foods to be tested are prepared in a way that they are typically consumed. For example, potatoes might be boiled, and bread might be toasted.
   - Each test food portion must contain exactly 50 grams of available carbohydrates. This means the portion size can vary depending on the carbohydrate content of the food.
3. **Baseline Measurement**
   - Participants fast overnight before the test to ensure a stable baseline for blood glucose levels.
   - On the test day, participants consume the test food in the morning.
4. **Blood Sample Collection**
   - Blood samples are taken at regular intervals over the next two hours to measure the blood glucose response. Typically, samples are taken at 15, 30, 45, 60, 90, and 120 minutes after consuming the food.

o The blood glucose levels are plotted on a graph to create a blood glucose response curve.

5. **Comparison with a Reference Food**
   o The blood glucose response of the test food is compared to that of a reference food, usually pure glucose or white bread, which is assigned a GI value of 100.
   o On separate occasions, participants consume the reference food, and blood glucose levels are measured in the same way as for the test food.

6. **Calculating the Glycemic Index**
   o The area under the blood glucose response curve (AUC) for both the test food and the reference food is calculated.
   o The GI value of the test food is determined by dividing the AUC for the test food by the AUC for the reference food and then multiplying by 100.

Factors Influencing GI Measurements

Several factors can influence the GI measurement of a food, including:

- **Ripeness:** Riper fruits tend to have higher GI values due to increased sugar content.
- **Cooking Methods:** Cooking can break down carbohydrates, making them more easily digestible and potentially raising the GI.
- **Food Processing:** Highly processed foods often have higher GI values because they are more quickly digested and absorbed.
- **Combination with Other Foods:** The presence of protein, fat, or fiber in a meal can slow down carbohydrate digestion and absorption, thereby lowering the overall GI of the meal.

Importance of Standardization

To ensure consistency and accuracy, it is crucial that GI testing follows standardized procedures, including:

- Using the same portion sizes of test and reference foods.
- Testing multiple participants to account for individual variations in blood glucose response.
- Conducting tests under controlled conditions, such as fasting and standardized blood sample collection times.

Understanding how the glycemic index is measured helps in appreciating its significance and reliability as a dietary tool. By incorporating low GI foods into their diet, individuals, particularly seniors, can better manage blood sugar levels, enhance overall health, and reduce the risk of chronic diseases.

1.3 Glycemic Index vs. Glycemic Load

Understanding both the glycemic index (GI) and glycemic load (GL) is crucial for making informed dietary choices, especially for seniors managing blood sugar levels. While the GI provides valuable insights into how quickly foods raise blood glucose levels, the GL offers a more comprehensive understanding by also considering the carbohydrate content of the food. This section explores the differences between these two concepts and their practical implications.

Glycemic Index (GI)

The glycemic index is a ranking system that measures how quickly carbohydrates in foods raise blood glucose levels compared to pure glucose. Foods are classified into three categories:

- **Low GI (55 or less):** Foods that cause a slow, gradual rise in blood glucose levels.
- **Medium GI (56 to 69):** Foods that cause a moderate increase in blood glucose levels.
- **High GI (70 or above):** Foods that cause a rapid spike in blood glucose levels.

While the GI is a useful tool for understanding the quality of carbohydrates, it does not consider the amount of carbohydrates consumed in a typical serving size. This is where the concept of glycemic load becomes important.

Practical Differences and Applications

1. Assessing Blood Sugar Impact:

- **GI Focus:** The GI primarily focuses on the rate at which carbohydrates raise blood glucose levels. For instance, watermelon has a high GI of 72, indicating it can quickly raise blood sugar levels.

- **GL Consideration:** Despite its high GI, watermelon has a low GL (around 4 per serving) because it contains relatively few carbohydrates per serving. This means a typical serving has a minimal impact on blood glucose levels.

2. Meal Planning:

- **GI Guidance:** Using the GI helps identify foods that cause rapid spikes in blood sugar, which is useful for planning low-GI meals.
- **GL Insight:** The GL provides a more comprehensive approach, allowing individuals to plan meals that consider both the type and amount of carbohydrates. For example, while a carrot has a high GI, its low carbohydrate content means its GL is low, making it a suitable choice for a low-GI meal plan.

3. Managing Chronic Conditions:

- **Diabetes Management:** For individuals with diabetes, both GI and GL are important. A food with a low GI but high carbohydrate content can still raise blood sugar levels significantly. Monitoring GL helps manage overall carbohydrate intake more effectively.
- **Heart Health and Weight Management:** Low GL diets are associated with reduced risks of cardiovascular diseases and better weight management. Incorporating low GL foods ensures balanced blood sugar levels and sustained energy without overconsumption of carbohydrates.

4. Overall Dietary Balance:

- **Balancing Nutrients:** The GI does not account for the nutritional content of foods other than carbohydrates. The GL provides a more holistic view, helping to balance the overall diet by considering the carbohydrate load along with other nutrients.

While the glycemic index is a useful tool for understanding how quickly carbohydrates in foods raise blood glucose levels, the glycemic load offers a more comprehensive picture by also considering the carbohydrate content of a typical serving. By using both GI and GL, seniors can make more informed dietary choices that support better blood sugar control, enhance overall health, and reduce the risk of chronic conditions. Incorporating low GI and low GL foods into the diet can help maintain stable blood glucose levels, support weight management, and improve heart health.

Chapter 2: Benefits of Low Glycemic Index Foods for Seniors

2.1 Blood Sugar Control

Managing blood sugar levels is crucial for maintaining overall health, particularly for seniors who may be at increased risk of diabetes and other related conditions. Understanding how the glycemic index (GI) and glycemic load (GL) of foods affect blood sugar can be instrumental in achieving better blood sugar control.

The Role of Blood Sugar Control

Blood sugar control refers to maintaining blood glucose levels within a target range, which is essential for preventing both short-term and long-term health complications. For seniors, effective blood sugar management can:

- **Prevent Diabetes:** Help prevent the onset of type 2 diabetes by maintaining normal blood glucose levels.
- **Reduce Complications:** Minimize the risk of diabetes-related complications such as neuropathy, retinopathy, and cardiovascular diseases.
- **Enhance Quality of Life:** Improve energy levels, cognitive function, and overall well-being.

How Low GI Foods Aid in Blood Sugar Control

Low glycemic index foods are those that cause a slow, gradual increase in blood glucose levels. Consuming low GI foods can have several beneficial effects on blood sugar control:

1. **Stable Blood Glucose Levels:**
   - Low GI food sources are processed and retained all the more leisurely, prompting a progressive arrival of glucose into the circulatory system. This helps prevent the sharp spikes and subsequent drops in blood sugar levels that can occur with high GI foods.
   - Stable blood glucose levels reduce the risk of hyperglycemia (high blood sugar) and hypoglycemia (low blood sugar), both of which can be harmful.

2. **Improved Insulin Sensitivity:**
   - Eating low GI foods can improve insulin sensitivity, meaning the body's cells are better able to respond to insulin and absorb glucose from the bloodstream. This is particularly important for seniors, as insulin sensitivity tends to decrease with age.
   - Enhanced insulin sensitivity helps in reducing insulin resistance, a key factor in the development of type 2 diabetes.

3. **Sustained Energy Levels:**
   - Low GI foods provide a slow and steady release of energy, which can help maintain consistent energy levels throughout the day. This is especially beneficial for seniors who may experience fatigue or energy dips with fluctuating blood sugar levels.
   - Consistent energy levels also support physical activity, which is crucial for overall health and blood sugar management.

4. **Reduced Risk of Overeating:**
   - Low GI foods tend to be more satiating, helping to control appetite and reduce the likelihood of overeating. This can aid in weight management, which is an important aspect of controlling blood sugar levels.
   - Maintaining a healthy weight is vital for reducing the risk of insulin resistance and type 2 diabetes.

Practical Tips for Blood Sugar Control with Low GI Foods

Incorporating low GI foods into your diet can significantly aid in blood sugar management. Here are a few functional tips for seniors:

1. **Choose Whole Grains:**
   - Opt for whole grains such as barley, quinoa, and oats instead of refined grains like white bread and rice. Whole grains have a lower GI and are rich in fiber, which slows down digestion and absorption.
2. **Incorporate High-Fiber Foods:**
   - Include plenty of high-fiber foods such as fruits, vegetables, legumes, and nuts. Fiber slows the release of glucose into the bloodstream, helping to maintain stable blood sugar levels.
3. **Combine Macronutrients:**
   - Pair carbohydrates with protein and healthy fats to slow the absorption of glucose. For example, have an apple with a handful of nuts or whole-grain toast with avocado and eggs.
4. **Monitor Portion Sizes:**
   - Indeed, even low GI food varieties can cause glucose spikes whenever ate in enormous amounts. Be aware of piece sizes and attempt to eat adjusted feasts.
5. **Stay Hydrated:**
   - Drinking plenty of water helps in maintaining blood sugar balance. Lack of hydration can prompt higher glucose levels.
6. **Regular Physical Activity:**
   - Take part in normal active work, like strolling, swimming, or yoga. Practice assists with bringing down blood glucose levels and further develops insulin responsiveness.

Effective blood sugar control is essential for seniors to maintain their health and prevent complications associated with diabetes. Incorporating low GI foods into the diet, along with mindful eating practices and regular physical activity, can significantly enhance blood sugar management. By understanding and utilizing the glycemic index, seniors can make informed dietary choices that support stable blood glucose levels and overall well-being.

2.2 Weight Management

Weight management is a crucial aspect of maintaining overall health, particularly for seniors. Managing weight effectively can help prevent chronic diseases, improve mobility, and enhance overall quality of life. Utilizing the glycemic index (GI) and glycemic load (GL) of foods can be an effective strategy for achieving and sustaining a healthy weight.

The Importance of Weight Management

Effective weight management is vital for several reasons:

- **Preventing Obesity:** Maintaining a healthy weight helps prevent obesity, which is associated with increased risks of diabetes, heart disease, and joint problems.
- **Improving Mobility:** A healthy weight reduces strain on the joints, which can improve mobility and physical function.
- **Enhancing Overall Health:** Proper weight management contributes to better control of blood pressure, cholesterol levels, and blood sugar levels, thereby reducing the risk of chronic diseases.

How Low GI Foods Aid in Weight Management

Incorporating low glycemic index foods into your diet can support weight management through several mechanisms:

1. **Increased Satiety and Reduced Hunger:**
   - Low GI foods are digested more slowly than high GI foods, leading to a gradual release of glucose into the bloodstream. This slow digestion helps keep you feeling full longer, reducing overall calorie intake.
   - For instance, foods like whole grains, legumes, and vegetables are low GI and tend to keep hunger at bay more effectively than high GI foods like sugary snacks.

2. **Stable Blood Sugar Levels:**
   - Low GI foods help maintain stable blood glucose levels, preventing the rapid spikes and crashes that can lead to increased appetite and cravings.
   - By avoiding the sharp increases in blood sugar that come with high GI foods, individuals are less likely to experience intense hunger or overeating.
3. **Improved Insulin Sensitivity:**
   - Low GI diets can improve insulin sensitivity, which is the body's ability to respond to insulin effectively. Better insulin sensitivity helps regulate blood sugar levels and can reduce fat storage.
   - Improved insulin sensitivity supports weight management by making it easier for the body to use glucose for energy rather than storing it as fat.
4. **Reduced Fat Storage:**
   - Consuming low GI foods can help lower insulin levels, which reduces the body's tendency to store excess glucose as fat.
   - Lower insulin levels make it easier for the body to burn stored fat for energy, aiding in weight loss and maintenance.

Practical Tips for Managing Weight with Low GI Foods

Implementing low GI foods into your diet can be an effective strategy for weight management. Here are some practical tips:

1. **Choose Whole Foods:**
   - Opt for whole, minimally processed foods with low GI values, such as vegetables, fruits, legumes, and whole grains. Examples include leafy greens, berries, lentils, and quinoa.
   - Whole foods provide essential nutrients and fiber, which support overall health and satiety.
2. **Pair Carbohydrates with Protein and Healthy Fats:**

- Combine low GI carbohydrates with protein and healthy fats to enhance satiety and reduce hunger. For example, pair a serving of whole-grain cereal with nuts or add avocado to a salad.
   - This combination helps maintain stable blood sugar levels and keeps you feeling full longer.

3. **Control Portion Sizes:**
   - Be mindful of portion sizes to avoid consuming excess calories, even from low GI foods. Pay attention to serving sizes and total calorie intake.
   - Using smaller plates and bowls can help manage portion sizes and prevent overeating.

4. **Plan Balanced Meals:**
   - Create meals that include a variety of low GI foods, such as a mixed vegetable stir-fry with brown rice and lean protein.
   - Balanced meals ensure a good mix of nutrients and help maintain stable blood sugar levels.

5. **Monitor and Adjust:**
   - Keep track of your food intake and how different foods affect your hunger and weight. Adjust your diet as needed based on your weight management goals and how your body responds.
   - Regularly review and update your eating plan to stay on track.

6. **Stay Active:**
   - Incorporate regular physical activity into your routine to complement a healthy diet. Exercise helps burn calories, improve metabolism, and support weight management.
   - Activities such as walking, swimming, or strength training can enhance overall health and weight control.

Effective weight management is essential for maintaining health and preventing chronic diseases, especially for seniors. By incorporating low GI foods into your diet, you can benefit from increased satiety, stable blood sugar levels, and improved insulin sensitivity. Combined with mindful portion control, balanced meals, and regular physical activity, these dietary strategies can support successful weight management and enhance overall quality of life.

2.3 Heart Health

Maintaining heart health is vital for overall well-being, especially as we age. Cardiovascular diseases, including heart disease and stroke, are leading causes of morbidity and mortality among seniors. Utilizing dietary strategies based on the glycemic index (GI) and glycemic load (GL) can play a significant role in supporting heart health and reducing the risk of cardiovascular conditions.

The Importance of Heart Health

Heart health is crucial for several reasons:

- **Reducing Risk of Cardiovascular Diseases:** Effective management of heart health can lower the risk of heart attacks, strokes, and other cardiovascular conditions.
- **Improving Blood Pressure:** Maintaining a healthy heart helps in managing blood pressure levels, reducing the risk of hypertension.
- **Enhancing Overall Quality of Life:** Good heart health contributes to better physical function, increased energy levels, and an improved quality of life.

How Low GI Foods Benefit Heart Health

Incorporating low glycemic index foods into your diet can positively impact heart health through several mechanisms:

1. **Lowering Blood Cholesterol Levels:**
   - Low GI foods are often rich in soluble fiber, which helps reduce low-density lipoprotein (LDL) cholesterol, commonly known as "bad" cholesterol. Examples include oats, beans, and apples.
   - Soluble fiber binds to cholesterol in the digestive tract and helps remove it from the body, contributing to lower overall cholesterol levels.

2. **Improving Blood Sugar Control:**
   - Low GI foods help maintain stable blood glucose levels, which is important for preventing insulin resistance and type 2 diabetes—conditions that are closely linked to cardiovascular diseases.
   - Consistent blood sugar control reduces the risk of developing diabetes-related complications, including heart disease.

3. **Reducing Inflammation:**
   - Many low GI foods are rich in antioxidants, vitamins, and minerals that help reduce inflammation. Persistent irritation is a gamble factor for cardiovascular illnesses.
   - Foods like fruits, vegetables, nuts, and whole grains contain anti-inflammatory compounds that contribute to heart health.

4. **Supporting Healthy Blood Pressure:**
   - A diet rich in low GI foods, particularly those high in potassium and magnesium, can help regulate blood pressure. Examples include leafy greens, bananas, and avocados.
   - Proper management of blood pressure is crucial for reducing the risk of heart disease and stroke.

Practical Tips for Supporting Heart Health with Low GI Foods

To support heart health effectively, consider incorporating these practical strategies:

1. **Prioritize Whole Grains:**
   - Choose whole grains like brown rice, quinoa, and barley over refined grains. Whole grains have lower GI values and are beneficial for heart health due to their fiber content.
   - Fiber-rich grains help lower cholesterol levels and support overall cardiovascular health.

2. **Incorporate Fruits and Vegetables:**
   - Include a variety of fruits and vegetables in your diet, focusing on those with low GI values. Berries, apples, and leafy greens are excellent choices.
   - These foods are rich in antioxidants and nutrients that help protect the heart and reduce inflammation.
3. **Select Lean Proteins:**
   - Settle on lean protein sources like fish, poultry, and vegetables. Fish, in particular, provides omega-3 fatty acids, which are known to reduce inflammation and lower the risk of heart disease.
   - Avoid processed meats and high-fat dairy products, which can negatively impact heart health.
4. **Use Healthy Fats:**
   - Consolidate solid fats from sources like nuts, seeds, avocados, and olive oil. These fats can help improve blood lipid profiles and support heart health.
   - Limit soaked and trans fats tracked down in seared food varieties, heated merchandise, and handled snacks.
5. **Monitor Sodium Intake:**
   - Reduce sodium intake by limiting the use of salt and avoiding processed foods high in sodium. Excess sodium can contribute to high blood pressure and increase cardiovascular risk.
   - Flavor foods with herbs and spices instead of salt to enhance taste without adding sodium.
6. **Stay Hydrated:**
   - Drink plenty of water to support overall cardiovascular health. Proper hydration helps maintain blood volume and supports heart function.
   - Limit sugary beverages and excessive caffeine, which can negatively impact heart health.

Supporting heart health is essential for overall well-being, especially for seniors. By incorporating low GI foods into your diet, you can benefit from improved cholesterol levels, better blood sugar control, reduced inflammation, and healthy blood pressure.

Combined with other heart-healthy practices such as choosing lean proteins, using healthy fats, and monitoring sodium intake, these dietary strategies can help reduce the risk of cardiovascular diseases and enhance overall quality of life.

2.4 Energy Levels and Mood

Maintaining stable energy levels and a positive mood is crucial for overall well-being, particularly as we age. The foods we consume have a significant impact on how energetic and emotionally balanced we feel. Understanding how the glycemic index (GI) and glycemic load (GL) of foods affect energy levels and mood can help in making dietary choices that support both physical and mental health.

The Impact of Diet on Energy Levels

Energy levels are influenced by how efficiently the body processes and utilizes the nutrients from food. Consuming foods with varying GI values can affect energy levels in the following ways:

1. **Stable Energy Release:**
   - Low GI foods provide a steady release of glucose into the bloodstream, leading to sustained energy levels throughout the day. Foods like whole grains, legumes, and vegetables are digested slowly, preventing rapid spikes and drops in blood sugar.
   - In contrast, high GI foods cause quick spikes in blood glucose, followed by rapid crashes that can lead to feelings of fatigue and low energy.

2. **Avoiding Energy Crashes:**
   - Eating high GI foods can lead to a surge in energy followed by a sharp decline as blood sugar levels drop. This fluctuation can cause feelings of tiredness and irritability.
   - By focusing on low GI foods, you can help maintain steady energy levels and avoid the energy crashes that often accompany high GI foods.

3. **Improved Physical Performance:**
   - Consuming low GI foods can improve physical endurance and performance by providing a more consistent supply of energy. This is particularly beneficial for engaging in daily activities and exercise.

The Connection Between Diet and Mood

Diet also plays a critical role in influencing mood and emotional well-being. The glycemic index and glycemic load of foods can impact mood in the following ways:

1. **Mood Stabilization:**
   - Low GI foods help stabilize blood sugar levels, which can contribute to a more balanced mood. Fluctuating blood glucose levels can lead to irritability, mood swings, and anxiety.
   - A steady supply of glucose from low GI foods supports brain function and emotional stability, helping to maintain a positive mood.
2. **Reducing Anxiety and Depression:**
   - Diets high in refined sugars and high GI foods have been linked to an increased risk of anxiety and depression. Low GI foods, with their steady impact on blood sugar levels, can help mitigate these risks.
   - Nutrient-dense low GI foods like fruits, vegetables, and whole grains contain vitamins and minerals that support brain health and mental well-being.
3. **Supporting Cognitive Function:**
   - Consuming low GI foods can support cognitive function by providing a consistent source of energy to the brain. Stable blood glucose levels help maintain focus, memory, and overall cognitive performance.

Maintaining stable energy levels and a positive mood is essential for overall well-being. By incorporating low glycemic index foods into your diet, you can support sustained energy release, stabilize blood sugar levels, and enhance emotional balance. Combined with regular hydration, balanced meals, and nutrient-rich foods, these dietary strategies can contribute to better energy levels, improved mood, and overall quality of life.

Chapter 3: Factors Affecting Glycemic Index

3.1 Types of Carbohydrates

Carbohydrates are one of the primary macronutrients essential for human health, providing the body with energy. They are found in a variety of foods, and their types can significantly influence health outcomes, particularly in terms of blood sugar control and energy levels. Understanding the different types of carbohydrates is crucial for making informed dietary choices, especially for seniors managing their glycemic index (GI) and glycemic load (GL).

Types of Carbohydrates

Carbs can be comprehensively arranged into three primary sorts: sugars, starches, and fiber. Each type has distinct characteristics and impacts on health.

1. **Sugars:**
   - **Monosaccharides:** These are the least complex type of starches and incorporate glucose, fructose, and galactose. They are single sugar molecules that are quickly absorbed by the body, leading to rapid increases in blood glucose levels.
     - *Examples:* Glucose is found in fruits and honey; fructose is also present in fruits and honey; galactose is found in dairy products.
   - **Disaccharides:** These consist of two monosaccharide molecules bonded together. atoms fortified together. Normal disaccharides incorporate sucrose (table sugar), lactose (milk sugar), and maltose (malt sugar).
     - *Examples:* Sucrose is found in sugar cane and sugar beets; lactose is found in milk and dairy products; maltose is found in germinating grains and malted beverages.

2. **Starches:**
   - **Polysaccharides:** These are complex carbohydrates composed of long chains of glucose molecules. They take longer to digest and absorb, resulting in a slower, more gradual release of glucose into the bloodstream.
     - *Examples:* Starchy foods include potatoes, corn, peas, and grains like rice, wheat, and oats.
   - **Amylose and Amylopectin:** Starches are made up of two types of molecules: amylose, which is a straight chain, and amylopectin, which is branched. Amylose tends to be digested more slowly, contributing to a lower GI, while amylopectin is digested more rapidly.

3. **Fiber:**
   - **Soluble Fiber:** This kind of fiber breaks up in water to shape a gel-like substance. It can help lower blood glucose and cholesterol levels. Soluble fiber slows down digestion and the absorption of glucose, leading to more stable blood sugar levels.
     - *Examples:* Soluble fiber is found in oats, barley, fruits (such as apples and citrus), legumes, and some vegetables.
   - **Insoluble Fiber:** This type of fiber does not dissolve in water and helps add bulk to the stool, promoting regular bowel movements. Insoluble fiber supports processing and can assist with forestalling obstruction.
     - *Examples:* Insoluble fiber is found in whole grains, nuts, seeds, and the skins of fruits and vegetables.

Impact of Carbohydrates on Blood Sugar and GI

The type of carbohydrate consumed can significantly impact blood sugar levels and the glycemic index of foods:

- **Simple Carbohydrates (Sugars):** These are quickly absorbed and can cause rapid spikes in blood sugar levels. High GI foods typically contain simple carbohydrates.
- **Complex Carbohydrates (Starches and Fiber):** These are digested more slowly, resulting in a gradual release of glucose and more stable blood sugar levels. Low GI foods usually contain complex carbohydrates, particularly those high in fiber.

Practical Tips for Choosing Carbohydrates

1. **Opt for Whole Foods:**
   - Choose whole, minimally processed foods that contain complex carbohydrates and fiber, such as whole grains, fruits, vegetables, and legumes.
2. **Limit Added Sugars:**
   - Reduce the intake of foods and beverages high in added sugars, such as sugary drinks, candies, and baked goods. These foods tend to have a high GI and can lead to rapid spikes in blood sugar.
3. **Incorporate Fiber-Rich Foods:**
   - Include a variety of fiber-rich foods in your diet to help regulate blood sugar levels and support digestive health. Aim for both soluble and insoluble fiber sources.
4. **Balance Carbohydrate Intake:**
   - Pair carbohydrates with protein and healthy fats to slow down the digestion process and provide a steady source of energy. For example, combine whole grain bread with avocado and lean protein.
5. **Monitor Portion Sizes:**
   - Be mindful of portion sizes, even for low GI foods, to avoid overconsumption of calories and maintain balanced blood sugar levels.

Understanding the different types of carbohydrates—sugars, starches, and fiber—and their impacts on blood sugar and overall health is crucial for making informed dietary choices. By prioritizing whole, complex carbohydrates and incorporating a variety of fiber-rich foods, seniors can better manage their glycemic index, support stable blood sugar levels, and promote overall health and well-being.

3.2 Fiber Content

Fiber is an essential component of a healthy diet, particularly for seniors. It plays a crucial role in maintaining digestive health, managing blood sugar levels, and supporting overall well-being. Understanding the different types of fiber and their benefits can help in making informed dietary choices that contribute to better health outcomes.

Types of Fiber

Fiber is a type of carbohydrate that the body cannot digest. It is sorted into two primary sorts: solvent and insoluble fiber. Both types offer distinct health benefits.

1. **Soluble Fiber:**
   - **Definition:** Solvent fiber disintegrates in water to shape a gel-like substance. It slows down digestion and can help control blood sugar levels and lower cholesterol.
   - **Sources:** Soluble fiber is found in oats, barley, nuts, seeds, beans, lentils, peas, and some fruits and vegetables, such as apples, citrus fruits, and carrots.
2. **Insoluble Fiber:**
   - **Definition:** Insoluble fiber does not dissolve in water. It adds mass to the stool and assists food with going all the more rapidly through the stomach and digestive organs.
   - **Sources:** Insoluble fiber is found in whole grains, nuts, beans, and vegetables such as cauliflower, green beans, and potatoes.

Health Benefits of Fiber

Incorporating fiber-rich foods into the diet offers numerous health benefits, especially for seniors:

1. **Improved Digestive Health:**
   - **Regular Bowel Movements:** Insoluble fiber helps promote regular bowel movements and prevent constipation by adding bulk to the stool.
   - **Healthy Gut Microbiome:** Fiber acts as a prebiotic, feeding the beneficial bacteria in the gut, which is essential for a healthy digestive system.
2. **Blood Sugar Control:**
   - **Stabilizing Blood Glucose Levels:** Soluble fiber slows the absorption of sugar, helping to stabilize blood glucose levels and reduce the risk of type 2 diabetes.
   - **Lower Glycemic Index:** Foods high in fiber typically have a lower glycemic index, meaning they cause a slower, more gradual increase in blood sugar levels.
3. **Heart Health:**
   - **Lowering Cholesterol Levels:** Soluble fiber binds to cholesterol particles in the digestive system and helps remove them from the body, lowering overall cholesterol levels and reducing the risk of heart disease.
   - **Reduced Blood Pressure:** High-fiber diets can help lower blood pressure, contributing to improved cardiovascular health.
4. **Weight Management:**
   - **Increased Satiety:** Fiber-rich foods are more filling and can help control appetite, leading to reduced calorie intake and supporting weight management.
   - **Healthy Weight Maintenance:** Maintaining a healthy weight is crucial for overall health, particularly for seniors, and a high-fiber diet can be an effective part of a weight management strategy.
5. **Reduced Risk of Chronic Diseases:**
   - **Prevention of Certain Cancers:** High-fiber diets have been associated with a reduced risk of certain types of cancer, particularly colorectal cancer.

- **Lowered Inflammation:** Fiber can help reduce inflammation in the body, which is linked to many chronic diseases, including heart disease, diabetes, and cancer.

Fiber is a vital component of a healthy diet, offering numerous benefits for digestive health, blood sugar control, heart health, weight management, and the prevention of chronic diseases. By incorporating a variety of fiber-rich foods, such as whole grains, fruits, vegetables, legumes, nuts, and seeds, seniors can enhance their overall health and well-being. Making informed dietary choices and increasing fiber intake can lead to improved health outcomes and a better quality of life.

3.3 Ripeness and Processing

The ripeness of foods and the degree of processing they undergo can significantly affect their glycemic index (GI) and overall nutritional value. Understanding these factors can help seniors make informed dietary choices that support better blood sugar control and overall health.

Ripeness

The ripeness of fruits and vegetables can influence their carbohydrate content and glycemic index. As fruits and vegetables ripen, their starches convert to sugars, which can increase their GI.

1. **Effect of Ripeness on Glycemic Index:**
   - **Increased Sugar Content:** As fruits ripen, their natural starches break down into simpler sugars such as glucose and fructose. This increases the fruit's sweetness and raises its GI.
     - *Examples:* A green, unripe banana has more starch and a lower GI compared to a fully ripe banana, which is higher in sugars and has a higher GI.
   - **Impact on Blood Sugar Levels:** Consuming riper fruits can cause a quicker spike in blood sugar levels due to the higher sugar content. For better blood sugar control, choosing slightly less ripe fruits may be beneficial.
2. **Nutritional Changes with Ripeness:**
   - **Vitamin and Antioxidant Levels:** The ripeness of fruits and vegetables can also affect their nutrient content. For example, some vitamins and antioxidants increase as the fruit ripens, potentially offering additional health benefits.

- *Examples:* Tomatoes and bell peppers may have higher levels of antioxidants like lycopene and vitamin C when fully ripe.
  - **Taste and Digestibility:** Ripe fruits and vegetables are generally sweeter and softer, which may be more palatable and easier to digest for some individuals, including seniors.

Processing

The processing of foods can significantly alter their glycemic index, fiber content, and overall nutritional value. Highly processed foods often have higher GIs and lower nutritional quality compared to minimally processed or whole foods.

1. **Impact of Processing on Glycemic Index:**
   - **Increased GI in Processed Foods:** Processing methods such as refining, grinding, and cooking can increase the GI of foods by breaking down their structure and making their carbohydrates more easily digestible.
     - *Examples:* Whole grains have a lower GI compared to their refined counterparts. For instance, whole grain bread has a lower GI than white bread.
   - **Reduction in Fiber:** Processing can remove fiber from foods, which raises their GI and reduces their ability to stabilize blood sugar levels.
     - *Examples:* Whole wheat flour contains more fiber and has a lower GI than white flour, which has had the bran and germ removed.
2. **Nutritional Changes with Processing:**
   - **Loss of Nutrients:** Processing can lead to a loss of essential nutrients such as vitamins, minerals, and antioxidants. Foods that are highly processed often have lower nutritional value.
     - *Examples:* Fresh fruits and vegetables generally contain more vitamins and antioxidants than canned or frozen versions, especially if the latter contain added sugars or preservatives.

- ○ **Addition of Unhealthy Ingredients:** Processed foods often contain added sugars, unhealthy fats, and sodium, which can negatively impact health.
  - *Examples:* Packaged snacks, sugary cereals, and fast foods are often high in added sugars and unhealthy fats, contributing to higher GIs and poorer overall nutrition.

3. **Minimally Processed Foods:**
   - ○ **Benefits of Minimal Processing:** Minimally processed foods, such as fresh fruits and vegetables, whole grains, and legumes, retain most of their natural nutrients and have lower GIs compared to highly processed foods.
     - *Examples:* Fresh apples, brown rice, and cooked lentils are minimally processed and provide more health benefits than their highly processed counterparts, such as apple juice, white rice, and canned lentil soup with added sodium.

The ripeness and processing of foods significantly impact their glycemic index and nutritional value. By understanding these factors, seniors can make better dietary choices that support stable blood sugar levels and overall health. Prioritizing less ripe fruits, whole grains, and minimally processed foods while limiting highly processed items can contribute to a balanced, nutrient-rich diet.

3.4 Cooking Methods

The way foods are cooked can have a significant impact on their glycemic index (GI) and overall nutritional value. Different cooking methods can alter the structure of carbohydrates, affect nutrient retention, and influence the rate at which foods are digested and absorbed. Understanding how various cooking methods impact the GI and nutritional content of foods can help seniors make informed dietary choices that support blood sugar control and overall health.

Impact of Cooking on Glycemic Index

Cooking can change the GI of foods by breaking down starches and fibers, making them more easily digestible. This can lead to higher or lower GI values depending on the cooking method used.

1. **Boiling and Steaming:**
    - **Lower GI:** Boiling and steaming can help retain the structure of carbohydrates, leading to a slower release of glucose into the bloodstream. These methods are generally gentle on the food and help preserve its fiber content.
        - *Examples:* Boiled or steamed vegetables, such as carrots and broccoli, typically have a lower GI compared to their roasted or fried counterparts.
    - **Nutrient Retention:** These methods also help preserve water-soluble vitamins, such as vitamin C and B vitamins, which can be lost during more intense cooking processes.
2. **Baking and Roasting:**
    - **Moderate GI:** Baking and roasting can increase the GI of certain foods by breaking down their starches and making them more easily digestible. However, these methods also caramelize the natural sugars in foods, which can enhance their flavor without adding extra sugar.

- ■ *Examples:* Baked potatoes have a higher GI than boiled potatoes, while roasted vegetables may have a slightly higher GI than steamed vegetables.
  - **Nutrient Impact:** While baking and roasting can lead to some nutrient loss, they generally preserve more nutrients than frying. Roasting vegetables can enhance their flavor and texture, making them more appealing.

3. **Frying:**
   - **Higher GI:** Frying foods can significantly increase their GI due to the breakdown of starches and the addition of fat. Fried foods are digested more quickly, leading to rapid spikes in blood sugar levels.
     - ■ *Examples:* Fried potatoes (such as French fries) have a higher GI compared to boiled or baked potatoes.
   - **Nutrient Loss:** Frying can lead to the loss of some vitamins and minerals, particularly if the food is fried at high temperatures. It also adds unhealthy fats, which can contribute to increased calorie intake and adverse health effects.

4. **Grilling and Broiling:**
   - **Variable GI:** Grilling and broiling can have varying effects on the GI of foods, depending on the type of food and how it is cooked. These methods can increase the GI of some foods by breaking down their starches, but they can also help retain nutrients and add flavor.
     - ■ *Examples:* Grilled vegetables may have a slightly higher GI than steamed vegetables, but they retain a lot of their nutritional value.
   - **Health Considerations:** Grilling and broiling are generally healthier cooking methods compared to frying, as they do not add extra fats. However, it's important to avoid charring the food, as this can produce harmful compounds.

5. **Microwaving:**
   - **Lower to Moderate GI:** Microwaving is a quick and convenient method that can help retain the nutritional content of foods while keeping the GI relatively low. It uses minimal water and short cooking times, which helps preserve vitamins and minerals.
     - *Examples:* Microwaved vegetables and grains can have a similar GI to their steamed or boiled counterparts.
   - **Nutrient Retention:** Microwaving is effective at preserving the nutrient content of foods, especially water-soluble vitamins that are prone to loss during longer cooking processes.

Practical Tips for Cooking Low GI Meals

1. **Use Gentle Cooking Methods:**
   - Prioritize gentle cooking methods such as steaming, boiling, and microwaving to maintain a lower GI and preserve the nutritional content of foods.

2. **Avoid Overcooking:**
   - Overcooking can break down the structure of foods, increasing their GI. Cook vegetables until they are just tender and grains until they are al dente.

3. **Combine Cooking Methods:**
   - Combine different cooking methods to balance flavor and nutrition. For example, lightly steam vegetables and then quickly roast them to add flavor while keeping the GI low.

4. **Limit Added Fats:**
   - Avoid cooking methods that require a lot of added fats, such as deep frying. Instead, use healthy fats like olive oil in moderation when roasting or grilling.

5. **Choose Whole Foods:**
   - Cook with whole, minimally processed ingredients to maintain a lower GI and higher nutritional value. Whole grains, fresh vegetables, and lean proteins should be staples in your cooking.
6. **Monitor Portion Sizes:**
   - Be mindful of portion sizes, even when using low GI foods and healthy cooking methods, to avoid excessive calorie intake and maintain balanced blood sugar levels.

Cooking methods can significantly influence the glycemic index and nutritional value of foods. By understanding the effects of different cooking techniques, seniors can make better dietary choices that support stable blood sugar levels and overall health. Prioritizing gentle cooking methods such as steaming, boiling, and microwaving, while avoiding excessive fats and overcooking, can help maintain the benefits of low GI foods and preserve essential nutrients.

3.5 Combination with Other Foods

Combining foods thoughtfully can significantly influence the glycemic index (GI) of a meal and its overall impact on blood sugar levels. By pairing high-GI foods with low-GI foods and incorporating macronutrients like proteins and fats, seniors can create balanced meals that promote stable blood sugar levels and provide essential nutrients for overall health.

Impact of Food Combinations on Glycemic Index

Combining different types of foods can moderate the glycemic impact of a meal. Here are some key principles and examples of how food combinations can affect the GI:

1. **Pairing High-GI Foods with Low-GI Foods:**
   - **Balancing Blood Sugar:** When high-GI foods are eaten with low-GI foods, the overall GI of the meal is reduced. This helps prevent rapid spikes in blood sugar levels and promotes more gradual increases.
     - *Examples:* Combining white rice (high-GI) with lentils or chickpeas (low-GI) creates a balanced meal with a moderate GI.
2. **Including Protein-Rich Foods:**
   - **Slowing Digestion:** Proteins take longer to digest than carbohydrates, which can slow down the absorption of glucose and moderate blood sugar levels.
     - *Examples:* Adding grilled chicken or tofu to a salad with high-GI ingredients like croutons or sweetened dressing can lower the overall GI of the meal.
3. **Incorporating Healthy Fats:**
   - **Enhancing Satiety:** Fats slow the digestive process, which helps stabilize blood sugar levels and keeps you feeling full for longer.
     - *Examples:* Drizzling olive oil on vegetables or adding avocado to a sandwich with high-GI bread can lower the meal's GI.

4. **Adding Fiber-Rich Foods:**
   - **Promoting Gradual Glucose Release:** Fiber slows down digestion and the absorption of glucose, resulting in more stable blood sugar levels.
     - *Examples:* Pairing a piece of fruit (high-GI) with a handful of nuts (fiber and fat) reduces the overall GI impact.
5. **Combining Different Types of Carbohydrates:**
   - **Moderating Glycemic Response:** Mixing high-GI and low-GI carbohydrates can lead to a more balanced glycemic response.
     - *Examples:* Eating pasta (moderate GI) with a variety of vegetables (low-GI) can create a meal with a balanced glycemic effect.

Combining different types of foods in a meal can significantly influence its glycemic index and overall impact on blood sugar levels. By pairing high-GI foods with low-GI foods, incorporating proteins and healthy fats, and including fiber-rich vegetables, seniors can create balanced meals that promote stable blood sugar levels and support overall health. Making thoughtful food combinations is a practical and effective strategy for managing glycemic responses and enhancing nutritional intake.

Chapter 4: Detailed Glycemic Index Food Charts

4.1 Fruits

4.1.1 High GI Fruits

Fruits are an essential part of a healthy diet, providing vital vitamins, minerals, fiber, and antioxidants. However, not all fruits have the same impact on blood sugar levels. High glycemic index (GI) fruits can cause rapid spikes in blood glucose, which can be a concern for seniors managing diabetes or other conditions that affect blood sugar control. Understanding which fruits fall into the high GI category and how to consume them mindfully can help seniors maintain better blood sugar control.

Characteristics of High GI Fruits

High GI fruits typically contain higher amounts of simple sugars and less fiber compared to their low GI counterparts. The glycemic index of these fruits is generally above 70 on the GI scale, which means they cause a more rapid increase in blood glucose levels.

Examples of High GI Fruits

1. **Watermelon:**
   - **GI Score:** Approximately 72
   - **Nutritional Benefits:** Watermelon is hydrating and rich in vitamins A and C, as well as antioxidants like lycopene.
   - **Considerations:** Due to its high water content, the actual glycemic load (GL) per serving is lower than some other high GI fruits, but it can still impact blood sugar levels if consumed in large quantities.

2. **Pineapple:**
   - **GI Score:** Approximately 66-70
   - **Nutritional Benefits:** Pineapple is a good source of vitamin C, manganese, and bromelain, an enzyme that aids digestion.
   - **Considerations:** Fresh pineapple has a higher GI than canned versions, especially if the canned pineapple is in juice or syrup.

3. **Ripe Bananas:**
   - **GI Score:** Approximately 62-72 (depending on ripeness)
   - **Nutritional Benefits:** Bananas are rich in potassium, vitamin B6, and fiber, especially when they are less ripe.
   - **Considerations:** The GI increases as bananas ripen. Opt for slightly green bananas to reduce the glycemic impact.

4. **Mango:**
   - **GI Score:** Approximately 51-60
   - **Nutritional Benefits:** Mangoes provide vitamins A and C, folate, and fiber.
   - **Considerations:** The GI of mangoes can vary depending on the variety and ripeness. Control is vital to dealing with its effect on glucose.

5. **Dates:**
   - **GI Score:** Approximately 42-103 (varies by type and ripeness)
   - **Nutritional Benefits:** Dates are high in fiber, potassium, and magnesium, making them a nutrient-dense option.
   - **Considerations:** Despite their high GI, dates have a moderate glycemic load when consumed in small quantities. They can be a good source of energy but should be eaten sparingly.

Managing High GI Fruits in the Diet

While high GI fruits can cause rapid increases in blood sugar levels, they can still be part of a balanced diet when consumed mindfully. Here are some tips for managing high GI fruits:

1. **Combine with Low GI Foods:**
   - Pair high GI fruits with foods that have a low GI to balance the overall glycemic impact of the meal.
     - *Examples:* Combine watermelon with a handful of nuts or pair pineapple with cottage cheese.
2. **Moderate Portion Sizes:**
   - Keep portion sizes small to minimize the impact on blood sugar levels.
     - *Examples:* Instead of a whole mango, have a few slices as part of a mixed fruit salad.
3. **Incorporate Protein and Healthy Fats:**
   - Adding protein and healthy fats to meals containing high GI fruits can slow down digestion and reduce blood sugar spikes.
     - *Examples:* Add sliced bananas to Greek yogurt with a sprinkle of chia seeds.
4. **Opt for Whole Fruits:**
   - Choose whole fruits over fruit juices or dried fruits, as whole fruits contain more fiber, which helps moderate the glycemic impact.
     - *Examples:* Eat fresh pineapple instead of drinking pineapple juice.
5. **Balance with Physical Activity:**
   - Physical activity can help regulate blood sugar levels. Consider going for a walk after consuming high GI fruits to help manage blood glucose levels.
6. **Monitor Blood Sugar Levels:**
   - Keep track of blood sugar levels before and after consuming high GI fruits to understand their impact and adjust portions and combinations as needed.

High GI fruits, such as watermelon, pineapple, ripe bananas, mango, and dates, can cause rapid increases in blood sugar levels. However, they can still be included in a healthy diet for seniors when consumed mindfully and in combination with low GI foods, proteins, and healthy fats. By managing portion sizes and incorporating physical activity, seniors can enjoy the nutritional benefits of these fruits while maintaining better blood sugar control.

4.1.2 Medium GI Fruits

Medium glycemic index (GI) fruits have a moderate impact on blood sugar levels, typically scoring between 56 and 69 on the GI scale. These fruits are a balanced choice for seniors who need to manage their blood sugar levels while still enjoying a variety of flavors and nutrients. Understanding the benefits and how to incorporate medium GI fruits into the diet can help seniors maintain a healthy, balanced diet.

Characteristics of Medium GI Fruits

Medium GI fruits generally contain a moderate amount of natural sugars and fiber. They provide a balanced release of glucose into the bloodstream, which helps prevent rapid spikes in blood sugar levels.

Examples of Medium GI Fruits

1. **Pineapple:**
   - **GI Score:** Approximately 56-66
   - **Nutritional Benefits:** Pineapple is rich in vitamin C, manganese, and the enzyme bromelain, which aids digestion.
   - **Considerations:** Fresh pineapple is a medium GI fruit, but its canned version, especially in syrup, can have a higher GI.
2. **Papaya:**
   - **GI Score:** Approximately 60
   - **Nutritional Benefits:** Papaya provides vitamins A and C, folate, and fiber. It likewise contains the catalyst papain, which helps absorption.
   - **Considerations:** Papaya is relatively low in calories and high in water content, making it a hydrating fruit option.
3. **Kiwi:**
   - **GI Score:** Approximately 50-58

- **Nutritional Benefits:** Kiwi is an excellent source of vitamin C, vitamin K, and fiber. It also contains antioxidants and has anti-inflammatory properties.
    - **Considerations:** The GI of kiwi can vary slightly depending on its ripeness. It is a nutrient-dense fruit that can be consumed in moderation.
4. **Oranges:**
    - **GI Score:** Approximately 43-53
    - **Nutritional Benefits:** Oranges are high in vitamin C, folate, and potassium. They also provide fiber, particularly when consumed with the pulp.
    - **Considerations:** Whole oranges have a lower GI compared to orange juice, which lacks fiber and can cause quicker spikes in blood sugar levels.
5. **Grapes:**
    - **GI Score:** Approximately 59
    - **Nutritional Benefits:** Grapes are a good source of vitamins C and K, as well as antioxidants such as resveratrol.
    - **Considerations:** Red and black grapes tend to have a lower GI compared to green grapes. Control is key because of their sugar content.

Managing Medium GI Fruits in the Diet

Medium GI fruits can be part of a balanced diet when consumed thoughtfully. Here are some tips for incorporating medium GI fruits into the diet of seniors:

1. **Pair with Low GI Foods:**
    - Combine medium GI fruits with low GI foods to create balanced meals and snacks.
        - *Examples:* Pair kiwi with a handful of almonds or add slices of orange to a spinach salad.
2. **Include Protein and Healthy Fats:**
    - Adding protein and healthy fats to meals with medium GI fruits can help slow digestion and stabilize blood sugar levels.

- *Examples:* Add slices of papaya to Greek yogurt or enjoy grapes with a piece of cheese.

3. **Monitor Portion Sizes:**
   - Keep portion sizes moderate to manage the glycemic impact and enjoy the nutritional benefits without causing blood sugar spikes.
     - *Examples:* A small bowl of pineapple chunks or a medium-sized orange can be a healthy, balanced snack.

4. **Incorporate Fiber-Rich Foods:**
   - Combine medium GI fruits with fiber-rich foods to enhance satiety and slow the release of glucose into the bloodstream.
     - *Examples:* Add kiwi to a bowl of oatmeal or top a whole grain cereal with slices of papaya.

5. **Opt for Whole Fruits:**
   - Choose whole fruits over fruit juices to benefit from the fiber content and lower GI.
     - *Examples:* Eat whole oranges instead of drinking orange juice or snack on whole grapes rather than consuming grape juice.

6. **Balance with Physical Activity:**
   - Physical activity can help manage blood sugar levels. Consider light exercise after consuming medium GI fruits to help regulate glucose levels.
     - *Examples:* A short walk after a meal with pineapple or a kiwi can help maintain stable blood sugar levels.

Example Meal Combinations

1. **Breakfast:**
   - **Balanced Smoothie:** Blend kiwi (medium GI) with spinach, Greek yogurt (protein), and a small amount of flaxseeds (healthy fats) for a balanced breakfast smoothie.

2. **Lunch:**
   - **Fruit and Nut Salad:** Mix orange slices (medium GI) with mixed greens, grilled chicken (protein), and a handful of walnuts (healthy fats) for a nutritious salad.
3. **Dinner:**
   - **Papaya Salsa:** Create a fresh salsa with diced papaya (medium GI), tomatoes, onions, cilantro, and lime juice, and serve it with grilled fish (protein).
4. **Snack:**
   - **Grapes and Cheese:** Enjoy a small bunch of grapes (medium GI) with a slice of cheese (protein and healthy fats) for a balanced snack.

Medium GI fruits like pineapple, papaya, kiwi, oranges, and grapes offer a balanced option for seniors looking to manage their blood sugar levels while enjoying a variety of nutritious and flavorful fruits. By combining these fruits with low GI foods, proteins, healthy fats, and fiber-rich options, seniors can create meals that promote stable blood sugar levels and provide essential nutrients. Moderation and mindful pairing can help seniors enjoy the benefits of medium GI fruits as part of a healthy, balanced diet.

4.1.3 Low GI Fruits

Low glycemic index (GI) fruits are an excellent choice for seniors who need to manage their blood sugar levels. These fruits have a GI score of 55 or lower, meaning they have a minimal impact on blood sugar levels, providing a steady and slow release of glucose into the bloodstream. Including low GI fruits in the diet can help maintain stable blood sugar levels, improve satiety, and contribute to overall health.

Characteristics of Low GI Fruits

Low GI fruits generally contain higher amounts of fiber, which slows the digestion and absorption of sugars. They also often have lower amounts of natural sugars compared to high or medium GI fruits.

Examples of Low GI Fruits

1. **Apples:**
    - **GI Score:** Approximately 36
    - **Nutritional Benefits:** Apples are rich in dietary fiber, particularly pectin, which aids digestion and helps regulate blood sugar levels. They also provide vitamins C and K and a variety of antioxidants.
    - **Considerations:** Eating apples with the skin on maximizes their fiber content and nutritional benefits.
2. **Berries (Strawberries, Blueberries, Raspberries):**
    - **GI Score:** Approximately 25-40
    - **Nutritional Benefits:** Berries are packed with vitamins C and K, fiber, and antioxidants like anthocyanins, which have anti-inflammatory and blood sugar-regulating properties.
    - **Considerations:** Fresh and frozen berries are both excellent choices. Avoid sweetened or canned versions to maintain their low GI benefits.
3. **Cherries:**
    - **GI Score:** Approximately 22

- ○ **Nutritional Benefits:** Cherries are high in antioxidants, including anthocyanins and vitamin C, and they provide a good amount of fiber.
  - ○ **Considerations:** Tart cherries have a slightly lower GI than sweet cherries and may offer additional anti-inflammatory benefits.

4. **Pears:**
   - ○ **GI Score:** Approximately 38
   - ○ **Nutritional Benefits:** Pears are a good source of dietary fiber, particularly when consumed with the skin. They also provide vitamins C and K and potassium.
   - ○ **Considerations:** Choose ripe but firm pears to maintain their fiber content and enjoy their low GI benefits.

5. **Plums:**
   - ○ **GI Score:** Approximately 24-53 (varies by variety and ripeness)
   - ○ **Nutritional Benefits:** Plums are rich in vitamins C and K, fiber, and antioxidants like phenolic compounds.
   - ○ **Considerations:** Consuming fresh plums rather than dried plums (prunes) helps maintain their lower GI.

6. **Grapefruit:**
   - ○ **GI Score:** Approximately 25
   - ○ **Nutritional Benefits:** Grapefruit is high in vitamins A and C and contains beneficial plant compounds like naringenin, which has antioxidant and anti-inflammatory properties.
   - ○ **Considerations:** Grapefruit can interact with certain medications, so it's important to consult with a healthcare provider if taking medications.

Managing Low GI Fruits in the Diet

Low GI fruits can be easily incorporated into a balanced diet for seniors. Here are some tips for maximizing their benefits:

1. **Pair with Protein and Healthy Fats:**
   - Combining low GI fruits with protein and healthy fats can further stabilize blood sugar levels and enhance satiety.
     - *Examples:* Add berries to a bowl of Greek yogurt or pair apple slices with almond butter.

2. **Include in Balanced Meals:**
   - Incorporate low GI fruits into meals to add flavor, nutrition, and fiber.
     - *Examples:* Add pear slices to a spinach salad with walnuts and feta cheese, or include cherries in a quinoa salad with mixed greens and goat cheese.

3. **Enjoy as Snacks:**
   - Low GI fruits make excellent snacks that provide a steady source of energy without causing blood sugar spikes.
     - *Examples:* Have a small bowl of mixed berries as a mid-morning snack or enjoy a plum with a handful of nuts in the afternoon.

4. **Use in Cooking and Baking:**
   - Low GI fruits can be used in a variety of recipes, adding natural sweetness and nutritional benefits.
     - *Examples:* Bake apples with a sprinkle of cinnamon for a healthy dessert or make a berry compote to top whole grain pancakes.

5. **Opt for Fresh or Frozen:**
   - Choose fresh or frozen fruits over canned or dried versions to maintain their low GI and maximize their nutritional value.
     - *Examples:* Fresh berries or frozen cherries can be added to smoothies or oatmeal.

Example Meal Combinations

1. **Breakfast:**
   - **Berry Smoothie:** Blend strawberries, blueberries (low GI), spinach, and a scoop of protein powder with unsweetened almond milk for a nutritious and balanced breakfast smoothie.
2. **Lunch:**
   - **Chicken and Pear Salad:** Mix sliced pears (low GI) with mixed greens, grilled chicken breast, walnuts, and a light vinaigrette for a satisfying lunch.
3. **Dinner:**
   - **Plum and Avocado Salsa:** Combine diced plums (low GI), avocado, red onion, cilantro, and lime juice to create a fresh salsa, and serve it with grilled fish.
4. **Snack:**
   - **Apple and Nut Butter:** Enjoy apple slices (low GI) with a tablespoon of almond butter for a balanced and satisfying snack.

Low GI fruits such as apples, berries, cherries, pears, plums, and grapefruit offer numerous health benefits while having a minimal impact on blood sugar levels. These fruits are rich in fiber, vitamins, antioxidants, and other essential nutrients, making them an excellent choice for seniors managing their blood sugar levels. By incorporating low GI fruits into meals, snacks, and recipes, seniors can enjoy their natural sweetness and nutritional benefits while maintaining stable blood sugar levels and overall health.

4.2 Vegetables

4.2.1 High GI Vegetables

While most vegetables are low on the glycemic index (GI), some starchy vegetables can have a high GI, which means they can cause a rapid increase in blood sugar levels. Understanding which vegetables fall into the high GI category and how to consume them in a balanced diet can help seniors manage their blood sugar levels more effectively.

Characteristics of High GI Vegetables

High GI vegetables generally contain more starch and less fiber compared to low GI vegetables. Their GI score is typically 70 or above, leading to quicker digestion and absorption of sugars, which can result in rapid spikes in blood glucose levels.

Examples of High GI Vegetables

1. **Potatoes:**
   - **GI Score:** Approximately 70-100 (varies by type and cooking method)
   - **Nutritional Benefits:** Potatoes are a good source of vitamins C and B6, potassium, and fiber (when consumed with the skin). They are also high in carbohydrates, which can lead to a high GI.
   - **Considerations:** The GI of potatoes varies based on their type and preparation. For example, baked or mashed potatoes have a higher GI compared to boiled or sweet potatoes.
2. **Parsnips:**
   - **GI Score:** Approximately 97
   - **Nutritional Benefits:** Parsnips provide vitamins C, E, K, and folate, as well as dietary fiber and antioxidants. They are, however, higher in natural sugars, contributing to their high GI.

- ○ **Considerations:** Cooking methods can influence the GI of parsnips. Roasting or mashing them can increase their glycemic impact.

3. **Pumpkin:**
   - ○ **GI Score:** Approximately 75
   - ○ **Nutritional Benefits:** Pumpkin is rich in vitamins A and C, potassium, and beta-carotene. It has a high water content and is low in calories but can have a high GI.
   - ○ **Considerations:** The GI of pumpkin can vary depending on the preparation. Roasting or mashing can increase its glycemic impact compared to boiling or steaming.

4. **Beets:**
   - ○ **GI Score:** Approximately 64 (boiled)
   - ○ **Nutritional Benefits:** Beets are high in folate, manganese, potassium, and antioxidants like betalains. Their natural sugars contribute to their higher GI.
   - ○ **Considerations:** Beets have a moderate to high GI when boiled, but the glycemic load remains moderate due to their fiber content.

Managing High GI Vegetables in the Diet

While high GI vegetables can cause rapid increases in blood sugar levels, they can still be included in a healthy diet when consumed mindfully. Here are some tips for managing high GI vegetables:

1. **Pair with Low GI Foods:**
   - ○ Combine high GI vegetables with low GI foods to balance the overall glycemic impact of the meal.
     - ■ *Examples:* Pair potatoes with non-starchy vegetables like broccoli or a leafy green salad.
2. **Include Protein and Healthy Fats:**
   - ○ Adding protein and healthy fats to meals containing high GI vegetables can slow down digestion and moderate blood sugar levels.

- *Examples:* Serve roasted parsnips with grilled chicken or fish, or add avocado to a pumpkin soup.

3. **Moderate Portion Sizes:**
   - Keep portion sizes small to minimize the impact on blood sugar levels.
     - *Examples:* Enjoy a small serving of mashed potatoes as a side dish rather than a main component of the meal.

4. **Opt for Less Processed Forms:**
   - Choose less processed forms of high GI vegetables to maintain more fiber and nutrients.
     - *Examples:* Eat boiled potatoes with the skin on instead of mashed potatoes, or choose fresh pumpkin over canned pumpkin.

5. **Balance with Physical Activity:**
   - Physical activity can help regulate blood sugar levels. Consider light exercise after consuming high GI vegetables to help manage blood glucose levels.
     - *Examples:* Take a short walk after a meal with parsnips or pumpkin.

Example Meal Combinations

1. **Breakfast:**
   - **Sweet Potato Hash:** Use sweet potatoes (lower GI than regular potatoes) mixed with spinach, bell peppers, and eggs for a balanced and nutritious breakfast.

2. **Lunch:**
   - **Beet Salad:** Combine boiled beets (moderate GI) with mixed greens, goat cheese, walnuts, and a vinaigrette for a nutritious salad that balances the glycemic impact.

3. **Dinner:**
   - **Pumpkin Soup:** Make a creamy pumpkin soup (moderate GI) with coconut milk and serve it with a side of grilled chicken or tofu for added protein.

4. **Snack:**

   ○ **Parsnip Chips:** Make baked parsnip chips (moderate portion) and pair them with a Greek yogurt dip for a balanced snack.

High GI vegetables like potatoes, parsnips, pumpkin, and beets can cause rapid increases in blood sugar levels, but they can still be part of a healthy diet when consumed thoughtfully. By pairing them with low GI foods, proteins, and healthy fats, and moderating portion sizes, seniors can enjoy the nutritional benefits of these vegetables while maintaining better blood sugar control. Understanding the glycemic impact of these vegetables and incorporating them wisely into meals can contribute to a balanced and healthful diet.

4.2.2 Medium GI Vegetables

Medium glycemic index (GI) vegetables have a moderate impact on blood sugar levels, typically scoring between 56 and 69 on the GI scale. These vegetables provide a balanced source of energy and nutrients without causing the rapid spikes in blood glucose associated with high GI foods. Incorporating medium GI vegetables into the diet can help seniors maintain stable blood sugar levels while enjoying a variety of flavors and textures.

Characteristics of Medium GI Vegetables

Medium GI vegetables contain moderate amounts of carbohydrates and fiber. They generally cause a gradual increase in blood sugar levels, providing a steady source of energy.

Examples of Medium GI Vegetables

1. **Carrots:**
   - **GI Score:** Approximately 41-49 (cooked)
   - **Nutritional Benefits:** Carrots are rich in beta-carotene, which the body converts to vitamin A. They also provide vitamins K, C, and fiber.
   - **Considerations:** The GI of carrots increases slightly when cooked, but they remain within the medium GI range.
2. **Corn:**
   - **GI Score:** Approximately 52-60
   - **Nutritional Benefits:** Corn is a good source of fiber, vitamins B and C, and essential minerals like magnesium and phosphorus.
   - **Considerations:** Fresh or frozen corn has a moderate GI. Avoid processed corn products like corn syrup, which have a much higher GI.
3. **Green Peas:**
   - **GI Score:** Approximately 48-54

- o **Nutritional Benefits:** Green peas are high in fiber, protein, vitamins A, C, K, and several B vitamins. They also contain various antioxidants.
  - o **Considerations:** Fresh or frozen peas are preferable over canned peas, which can have added sugars and salt.

4. **Sweet Potatoes:**
   - o **GI Score:** Approximately 63
   - o **Nutritional Benefits:** Sweet potatoes are rich in beta-carotene, vitamins C and B6, potassium, and fiber.
   - o **Considerations:** The GI of sweet potatoes can vary depending on the cooking method. Boiling results in a lower GI compared to baking or roasting.

5. **Butternut Squash:**
   - o **GI Score:** Approximately 51-65
   - o **Nutritional Benefits:** Butternut squash is a great source of vitamins A and C, fiber, and several important minerals like potassium and magnesium.
   - o **Considerations:** The GI of butternut squash can vary with preparation methods. Boiling or steaming results in a lower GI compared to roasting or mashing.

Managing Medium GI Vegetables in the Diet

Medium GI vegetables can be a valuable part of a balanced diet for seniors. Here are some tips for incorporating them into meals:

1. **Pair with Low GI Foods:**
   - o Combine medium GI vegetables with low GI foods to create balanced meals and moderate the overall glycemic impact.
     - *Examples:* Add green peas to a mixed vegetable stir-fry with broccoli and bell peppers.

2. **Include Protein and Healthy Fats:**
   - Adding protein and healthy fats to meals with medium GI vegetables can help stabilize blood sugar levels and enhance satiety.
     - *Examples:* Serve sweet potatoes with grilled chicken or add avocado to a corn and black bean salad.

3. **Monitor Portion Sizes:**
   - Keep portion sizes moderate to manage the glycemic impact while enjoying the nutritional benefits.
     - *Examples:* Enjoy a small serving of roasted butternut squash as a side dish.

4. **Opt for Whole Forms:**
   - Choose whole, unprocessed forms of medium GI vegetables to maintain their fiber content and nutritional value.
     - *Examples:* Eat fresh or frozen corn instead of processed corn products.

5. **Balance with Physical Activity:**
   - Physical activity can help regulate blood sugar levels. Light exercise after meals can be beneficial.
     - *Examples:* Take a walk after a meal that includes cooked carrots or sweet potatoes.

Example Meal Combinations

1. **Breakfast:**
   - **Sweet Potato Hash:** Combine diced sweet potatoes (medium GI) with spinach, bell peppers, and eggs for a nutritious and balanced breakfast.

2. **Lunch:**
   - **Butternut Squash Soup:** Make a creamy butternut squash soup (medium GI) with low-fat coconut milk and serve it with a side of mixed greens and grilled chicken.

3. **Dinner:**
   - **Pea and Carrot Stir-Fry:** Stir-fry green peas (medium GI) and carrots (medium GI) with tofu or shrimp, and serve over brown rice.
4. **Snack:**
   - **Corn Salad:** Mix fresh corn (medium GI) with diced tomatoes, red onion, cilantro, and a light lime vinaigrette for a refreshing snack.

Medium GI vegetables like carrots, corn, green peas, sweet potatoes, and butternut squash provide a moderate impact on blood sugar levels, making them a balanced choice for seniors. These vegetables are rich in essential nutrients, fiber, and antioxidants, contributing to overall health. By combining them with low GI foods, proteins, and healthy fats, and keeping portion sizes moderate, seniors can enjoy the benefits of these vegetables while maintaining stable blood sugar levels. Incorporating medium GI vegetables into a balanced diet can help seniors achieve better blood sugar control and improve their overall well-being.

6.2.3 Low GI Vegetables

Low glycemic index (GI) vegetables have a minimal impact on blood sugar levels, typically scoring 55 or below on the GI scale. These vegetables are a cornerstone of a healthy diet for seniors, offering numerous nutritional benefits without causing significant spikes in blood glucose. Including a variety of low GI vegetables in the diet can help seniors manage their blood sugar levels, enhance satiety, and promote overall health.

Characteristics of Low GI Vegetables

Low GI vegetables are generally high in fiber and water content and low in carbohydrates. They digest slowly, resulting in a gradual release of glucose into the bloodstream.

Examples of Low GI Vegetables

1. **Leafy Greens:**
    - **Examples:** Spinach, kale, Swiss chard, arugula
    - **GI Score:** Typically 10-15
    - **Nutritional Benefits:** Leafy greens are rich in vitamins A, C, K, and folate. They also provide important minerals like calcium and iron, and are high in fiber and antioxidants.
    - **Considerations:** Leafy greens can be consumed raw in salads, added to smoothies, or lightly sautéed for a nutrient-packed side dish.
2. **Broccoli:**
    - **GI Score:** Approximately 10-15
    - **Nutritional Benefits:** Broccoli is high in vitamins C and K, fiber, and antioxidants like sulforaphane, which has anti-cancer properties.
    - **Considerations:** Steaming or roasting broccoli retains its nutrients while keeping its GI low.

3. **Cauliflower:**
   - **GI Score:** Approximately 15-20
   - **Nutritional Benefits:** Cauliflower is a good source of vitamins C and K, fiber, and several B vitamins. It also contains compounds that support liver health.
   - **Considerations:** Cauliflower can be roasted, steamed, or mashed as a low-carb alternative to potatoes or rice.

4. **Zucchini:**
   - **GI Score:** Approximately 15
   - **Nutritional Benefits:** Zucchini is rich in vitamins A and C, potassium, and fiber. It is also low in calories and high in water content.
   - **Considerations:** Zucchini can be grilled, sautéed, or spiralized into noodles as a healthy pasta substitute.

5. **Bell Peppers:**
   - **GI Score:** Approximately 10-20
   - **Nutritional Benefits:** Bell peppers are high in vitamins A and C, fiber, and antioxidants like beta-carotene and lutein.
   - **Considerations:** Bell peppers can be eaten raw in salads, stuffed with grains and protein, or roasted for a sweet, caramelized flavor.

6. **Tomatoes:**
   - **GI Score:** Approximately 15
   - **Nutritional Benefits:** Tomatoes are rich in vitamins C and K, potassium, and the antioxidant lycopene, which supports heart health.
   - **Considerations:** Fresh tomatoes have a low GI. They can be used in salads, soups, sauces, or roasted for added flavor.

7. **Cucumbers:**
   - **GI Score:** Approximately 15
   - **Nutritional Benefits:** Cucumbers are high in water content, vitamins K and C, and fiber. They are also low in calories.

- **Considerations:** Cucumbers are best consumed fresh in salads or as a hydrating snack.

Managing Low GI Vegetables in the Diet

Low GI vegetables can be easily incorporated into a balanced diet for seniors. Here are some tips for maximizing their benefits:

1. **Incorporate into Every Meal:**
   - Include a variety of low GI vegetables in every meal to ensure a steady intake of essential nutrients and fiber.
     - *Examples:* Add spinach to breakfast smoothies, include a side salad with lunch, and serve steamed broccoli with dinner.
2. **Combine with Proteins and Healthy Fats:**
   - Pair low GI vegetables with proteins and healthy fats to create balanced and satisfying meals.
     - *Examples:* Add grilled chicken to a kale salad or top a stir-fry with tofu and sesame seeds.
3. **Use in Snacks:**
   - Low GI vegetables make excellent snacks that provide nutrients and fiber without spiking blood sugar levels.
     - *Examples:* Snack on cucumber slices with hummus or bell pepper strips with guacamole.
4. **Prepare in Different Ways:**
   - Experiment with different cooking methods to keep meals interesting and flavorful.
     - *Examples:* Roast cauliflower with spices, steam zucchini with garlic, or sauté bell peppers with onions.
5. **Include in Soups and Stews:**
   - Add low GI vegetables to soups and stews for a nutrient-dense, filling meal.

- *Examples:* Make a vegetable minestrone with tomatoes, zucchini, and spinach or a broccoli and cauliflower soup.

Example Meal Combinations

1. **Breakfast:**
   - **Green Smoothie:** Blend spinach (low GI), kale, a banana (moderate GI), and almond milk for a nutritious and filling breakfast smoothie.
2. **Lunch:**
   - **Stuffed Bell Peppers:** Fill bell peppers (low GI) with quinoa, black beans, corn, and salsa for a satisfying and balanced lunch.
3. **Dinner:**
   - **Vegetable Stir-Fry:** Stir-fry broccoli (low GI), zucchini (low GI), bell peppers (low GI), and tofu with a low-sodium soy sauce.
4. **Snack:**
   - **Cucumber and Hummus:** Enjoy cucumber slices (low GI) with a serving of hummus for a healthy, fiber-rich snack.

Low GI vegetables like leafy greens, broccoli, cauliflower, zucchini, bell peppers, tomatoes, and cucumbers offer numerous health benefits without significantly impacting blood sugar levels. These vegetables are rich in vitamins, minerals, fiber, and antioxidants, making them a valuable part of a balanced diet for seniors. By incorporating a variety of low GI vegetables into meals and snacks, seniors can enjoy their nutritional benefits while maintaining stable blood sugar levels and overall well-being.

4.3 Grains and Cereals

4.3.1 High GI Grains

High glycemic index (GI) grains are carbohydrates that break down quickly during digestion, causing a rapid increase in blood sugar levels. These grains typically have a GI score of 70 or above. While they can provide quick energy, frequent consumption of high GI grains can lead to spikes and crashes in blood sugar levels, which can be particularly problematic for seniors managing diabetes or other blood sugar-related conditions. Understanding the characteristics and examples of high GI grains can help seniors make informed dietary choices.

Characteristics of High GI Grains

High GI grains are often refined or processed, which removes fiber and other nutrients, resulting in faster digestion and absorption. These grains tend to have lower fiber content compared to their whole grain counterparts, contributing to their higher GI.

Examples of High GI Grains

1. **White Bread:**
    - **GI Score:** Approximately 70-85
    - **Nutritional Benefits:** White bread provides quick energy and some B vitamins and iron, but it is low in fiber and other essential nutrients.
    - **Considerations:** White bread is highly processed and has most of its fiber removed, leading to rapid spikes in blood sugar levels.
2. **White Rice:**
    - **GI Score:** Approximately 70-90
    - **Nutritional Benefits:** White rice provides quick energy and some B vitamins and minerals like magnesium, but it lacks fiber and has fewer nutrients compared to brown rice.

- Considerations: Opting for whole grain rice or alternatives like quinoa can help lower the GI of meals.

3. **Instant Oatmeal:**
   - **GI Score:** Approximately 70-75
   - **Nutritional Benefits:** Instant oatmeal provides some fiber and nutrients like iron and B vitamins, but it often has added sugars and less fiber than steel-cut or rolled oats.
   - **Considerations:** Choosing less processed forms of oats can reduce the GI and provide more sustained energy.

4. **Cornflakes:**
   - **GI Score:** Approximately 80-85
   - **Nutritional Benefits:** Cornflakes offer some vitamins and minerals, but they are typically low in fiber and high in added sugars.
   - **Considerations:** Whole grain cereals or those with higher fiber content are better options for stable blood sugar levels.

5. **Rice Cakes:**
   - **GI Score:** Approximately 70-80
   - **Nutritional Benefits:** Rice cakes are low in calories and provide quick energy, but they are also low in fiber and other nutrients.
   - **Considerations:** Pairing rice cakes with protein or healthy fats can help moderate their glycemic impact.

6. **Pretzels:**
   - **GI Score:** Approximately 80-85
   - **Nutritional Benefits:** Pretzels provide quick energy and some B vitamins, but they are low in fiber and high in sodium.
   - **Considerations:** Whole grain or higher fiber snacks can be better choices for blood sugar management.

Managing High GI Grains in the Diet

While high GI grains can cause rapid increases in blood sugar levels, they can still be included in the diet in moderation and when paired with other foods that help balance their impact. Here are some strategies for managing high GI grains:

1. **Pair with Low GI Foods:**
   - Combining high GI grains with low GI foods can help moderate the overall glycemic impact of the meal.
     - *Examples:* Pair white rice with a variety of non-starchy vegetables and lean protein.
2. **Add Fiber, Protein, and Healthy Fats:**
   - Including fiber, protein, and healthy fats in meals with high GI grains can slow down digestion and help stabilize blood sugar levels.
     - *Examples:* Top white bread with avocado and an egg for breakfast.
3. **Moderate Portion Sizes:**
   - Keeping portion sizes small can help manage the glycemic impact while still enjoying high GI grains occasionally.
     - *Examples:* Have a small serving of instant oatmeal with a handful of nuts and berries.
4. **Choose Whole Grain Alternatives:**
   - Opt for whole grain alternatives whenever possible to benefit from more fiber and nutrients.
     - *Examples:* Substitute white rice with brown rice or quinoa, or choose whole grain bread over white bread.
5. **Balance with Physical Activity:**
   - Engaging in physical activity after meals can help manage blood sugar levels.
     - *Examples:* Take a walk after eating a meal that includes high GI grains.

Example Meal Combinations

1. **Breakfast:**
   - **Whole Grain Toast with Avocado:** Replace white bread with whole grain toast and top with mashed avocado and a sprinkle of chia seeds for added fiber and healthy fats.
2. **Lunch:**
   - **Brown Rice and Vegetable Stir-Fry:** Swap white rice for brown rice and stir-fry with a mix of low GI vegetables like broccoli, bell peppers, and snap peas.
3. **Dinner:**
   - **Quinoa Salad:** Use quinoa instead of white rice in a salad with mixed greens, cherry tomatoes, cucumber, and grilled chicken for a balanced meal.
4. **Snack:**
   - **Greek Yogurt with Berries:** Choose Greek yogurt with fresh berries instead of cornflakes to add protein and fiber.

High GI grains like white bread, white rice, instant oatmeal, cornflakes, rice cakes, and pretzels can cause rapid increases in blood sugar levels. While these grains can provide quick energy, it is essential for seniors to consume them in moderation and pair them with low GI foods, fiber, protein, and healthy fats to help balance their glycemic impact. By making mindful choices and opting for whole grain alternatives, seniors can enjoy a variety of grains in their diet while maintaining stable blood sugar levels and overall health.

4.3.2 Medium GI Grains

Medium glycemic index (GI) grains have a moderate impact on blood sugar levels, with GI scores typically ranging from 56 to 69. These grains provide a balance between quick energy release and sustained energy, making them a suitable choice for seniors looking to manage their blood sugar levels while still enjoying a variety of grains in their diet. Including medium GI grains can contribute to a nutritious and balanced diet.

Characteristics of Medium GI Grains

Medium GI grains have a moderate amount of fiber and nutrients, which helps slow down digestion compared to high GI grains. They provide a steady source of energy without causing rapid spikes in blood glucose levels.

Examples of Medium GI Grains

1. **Brown Rice:**
   - **GI Score:** Approximately 50-55
   - **Nutritional Benefits:** Brown rice is a whole grain that retains its bran and germ, providing fiber, vitamins B1, B3, B6, and minerals like magnesium and phosphorus.
   - **Considerations:** Brown rice is a versatile grain that can be used in various dishes, providing a steady release of energy.
2. **Bulgar Wheat:**
   - **GI Score:** Approximately 48-58
   - **Nutritional Benefits:** Bulgar wheat is partially cooked and cracked wheat that retains most of its fiber and nutrients, including B vitamins and minerals like iron and magnesium.
   - **Considerations:** Bulgar wheat is commonly used in Mediterranean dishes like tabbouleh and can be a hearty addition to soups and salads.
3. **Basmati Rice:**
   - **GI Score:** Approximately 58-65

- **Nutritional Benefits:** Basmati rice is a long-grain rice that is lower in GI compared to regular white rice and provides some fiber, vitamins, and minerals.
  - **Considerations:** Basmati rice has a fragrant aroma and can be paired with a variety of dishes, particularly in Indian cuisine.

4. **Whole Wheat Pasta:**
   - **GI Score:** Approximately 55-60
   - **Nutritional Benefits:** Whole wheat pasta retains the bran and germ of the wheat, offering more fiber, protein, and nutrients like iron and magnesium compared to regular pasta.
   - **Considerations:** Whole wheat pasta can be a healthier alternative to refined pasta and pairs well with vegetables and lean proteins.

5. **Oatmeal (Rolled or Steel-Cut):**
   - **GI Score:** Approximately 55-60
   - **Nutritional Benefits:** Oatmeal is high in fiber, particularly beta-glucan, which helps with heart health and blood sugar control. It also provides vitamins B1 and B5, iron, and magnesium.
   - **Considerations:** Rolled or steel-cut oats have a lower GI compared to instant oats and can be a hearty breakfast option.

6. **Quinoa:**
   - **GI Score:** Approximately 53
   - **Nutritional Benefits:** Quinoa is a pseudo-grain that is high in protein, fiber, and essential amino acids. It also provides vitamins B and E, iron, magnesium, and potassium.
   - **Considerations:** Quinoa is gluten-free and can be used in salads, as a side dish, or as a base for grain bowls.

Managing Medium GI Grains in the Diet

Medium GI grains can be an excellent addition to a balanced diet for seniors. Here are some tips for incorporating them effectively:

1. **Pair with Low GI Foods:**
   - Combine medium GI grains with low GI foods to balance the overall glycemic impact of the meal.
     - *Examples:* Serve quinoa with a mix of leafy greens and grilled chicken.
2. **Include Protein and Healthy Fats:**
   - Adding protein and healthy fats to meals with medium GI grains can help stabilize blood sugar levels and enhance satiety.
     - *Examples:* Add nuts and seeds to oatmeal or top whole wheat pasta with a lean protein source.
3. **Monitor Portion Sizes:**
   - Keep portion sizes moderate to manage the glycemic impact while still benefiting from the nutritional content of the grains.
     - *Examples:* Have a small serving of brown rice alongside a larger portion of vegetables and protein.
4. **Use in Varied Recipes:**
   - Incorporate medium GI grains into a variety of recipes to keep meals interesting and nutritious.
     - *Examples:* Use bulgar wheat in a tabbouleh salad or basmati rice in a curry dish.
5. **Balance with Physical Activity:**
   - Physical activity can help regulate blood sugar levels. Consider light exercise after consuming medium GI grains.
     - *Examples:* Take a walk after a meal that includes brown rice or whole wheat pasta.

Example Meal Combinations

1. **Breakfast:**
   - **Oatmeal with Fruit and Nuts:** Prepare rolled or steel-cut oats and top with fresh berries, a handful of nuts, and a drizzle of honey for a balanced and satisfying breakfast.
2. **Lunch:**
   - **Quinoa Salad:** Combine cooked quinoa with mixed greens, cherry tomatoes, cucumber, avocado, and grilled chicken for a nutrient-dense salad.
3. **Dinner:**
   - **Whole Wheat Pasta Primavera:** Toss whole wheat pasta with sautéed vegetables like bell peppers, zucchini, and broccoli, and add a lean protein like shrimp or chicken.
4. **Snack:**
   - **Bulgar Wheat Tabbouleh:** Mix cooked bulgar wheat with parsley, mint, tomatoes, cucumber, and a lemon-olive oil dressing for a refreshing and fiber-rich snack.

Medium GI grains such as brown rice, bulgar wheat, basmati rice, whole wheat pasta, oatmeal, and quinoa provide a balanced source of energy and nutrients, making them a valuable part of a healthy diet for seniors. These grains offer more fiber and nutrients compared to high GI grains, helping to maintain stable blood sugar levels and promote overall health. By pairing medium GI grains with low GI foods, proteins, and healthy fats, and keeping portion sizes moderate, seniors can enjoy their nutritional benefits while managing their blood sugar levels effectively. Incorporating a variety of medium GI grains into the diet can enhance dietary diversity and contribute to long-term health and well-being.

4.3.3 Low GI Grains

Low glycemic index (GI) grains are those with a GI score of 55 or below, meaning they have a minimal impact on blood sugar levels. These grains digest slowly, providing a steady release of glucose into the bloodstream. Including low GI grains in the diet is especially beneficial for seniors, as they help maintain stable blood sugar levels, enhance satiety, and contribute to overall health.

Characteristics of Low GI Grains

Low GI grains are typically whole grains that retain their bran and germ, which are rich in fiber, vitamins, and minerals. The high fiber content slows down digestion and absorption, leading to a more gradual increase in blood sugar levels.

Examples of Low GI Grains

1. **Barley:**
   - **GI Score:** Approximately 28
   - **Nutritional Benefits:** Barley is high in fiber, particularly beta-glucan, which helps lower cholesterol levels. It also provides vitamins B1, B3, B6, and minerals such as selenium, magnesium, and phosphorus.
   - **Considerations:** Barley can be used in soups, stews, salads, and as a rice substitute.
2. **Whole Grain Bread:**
   - **GI Score:** Approximately 51
   - **Nutritional Benefits:** Whole grain bread retains the bran and germ, providing more fiber, protein, and nutrients like iron, magnesium, and zinc compared to white bread.
   - **Considerations:** Look for bread made from 100% whole grains without added sugars.
3. **Steel-Cut Oats:**
   - **GI Score:** Approximately 42

- ○ **Nutritional Benefits:** Steel-cut oats are less processed than rolled or instant oats, preserving more fiber and nutrients. They are rich in beta-glucan, which supports heart health and blood sugar control.
- ○ **Considerations:** Steel-cut oats take longer to cook but provide a chewy texture and nutty flavor.

4. **Quinoa:**
   - ○ **GI Score:** Approximately 53
   - ○ **Nutritional Benefits:** Quinoa is a pseudo-grain high in protein, fiber, and essential amino acids. It also offers vitamins B and E, iron, magnesium, and potassium.
   - ○ **Considerations:** Quinoa is gluten-free and versatile, suitable for salads, side dishes, and grain bowls.

5. **Buckwheat:**
   - ○ **GI Score:** Approximately 49
   - ○ **Nutritional Benefits:** Buckwheat is rich in fiber, protein, and essential amino acids. It also contains antioxidants like rutin and quercetin, and minerals such as magnesium and copper.
   - ○ **Considerations:** Buckwheat can be used in porridge, pancakes, or as a rice substitute.

6. **Freekeh:**
   - ○ **GI Score:** Approximately 43
   - ○ **Nutritional Benefits:** Freekeh is a young green wheat harvested early and roasted. It is high in fiber, protein, and nutrients like magnesium, zinc, and iron.
   - ○ **Considerations:** Freekeh has a nutty, slightly smoky flavor and can be used in salads, pilafs, and as a side dish.

Managing Low GI Grains in the Diet

Low GI grains can be easily incorporated into a balanced diet for seniors. Here are some tips for maximizing their benefits:

1. **Incorporate into Every Meal:**
   - Include a variety of low GI grains in each meal to ensure a steady intake of essential nutrients and fiber.
     - *Examples:* Have steel-cut oats for breakfast, a quinoa salad for lunch, and barley soup for dinner.

2. **Pair with Proteins and Healthy Fats:**
   - Combining low GI grains with proteins and healthy fats can further stabilize blood sugar levels and enhance satiety.
     - *Examples:* Top quinoa with grilled chicken and avocado, or add nuts and seeds to oatmeal.

3. **Use in Diverse Recipes:**
   - Incorporate low GI grains into a variety of recipes to keep meals interesting and flavorful.
     - *Examples:* Use freekeh in a grain bowl, make buckwheat pancakes, or add barley to a vegetable soup.

4. **Balance with Vegetables and Legumes:**
   - Combining low GI grains with vegetables and legumes can create nutrient-dense and balanced meals.
     - *Examples:* Pair whole grain bread with a lentil and vegetable soup or serve a barley salad with mixed greens.

5. **Monitor Portion Sizes:**
   - While low GI grains are beneficial, it's important to keep portion sizes moderate to manage overall caloric intake.
     - *Examples:* Enjoy a moderate serving of quinoa alongside a larger portion of non-starchy vegetables.

Example Meal Combinations

1. **Breakfast:**
   - **Steel-Cut Oats with Berries:** Cook steel-cut oats and top with fresh berries, a sprinkle of nuts, and a drizzle of honey for a nutritious and filling breakfast.
2. **Lunch:**
   - **Quinoa and Black Bean Salad:** Combine cooked quinoa with black beans, corn, cherry tomatoes, avocado, and a lime vinaigrette for a protein-rich and satisfying salad.
3. **Dinner:**
   - **Barley and Vegetable Soup:** Make a hearty soup with barley, carrots, celery, onions, and spinach, seasoned with herbs and spices.
4. **Snack:**
   - **Whole Grain Bread with Hummus:** Spread hummus on slices of whole grain bread for a fiber-rich and protein-packed snack.

Low GI grains such as barley, whole grain bread, steel-cut oats, quinoa, buckwheat, and freekeh offer numerous health benefits for seniors. These grains are high in fiber, vitamins, minerals, and antioxidants, which contribute to stable blood sugar levels, enhanced satiety, and overall well-being. By incorporating a variety of low GI grains into meals and pairing them with proteins, healthy fats, and vegetables, seniors can enjoy their nutritional advantages while maintaining stable blood sugar levels and promoting long-term health.

4.4 Dairy and Alternatives

4.4.1 High GI Dairy Products

Dairy products are generally known for their low glycemic index (GI) due to their protein and fat content, which slows down carbohydrate absorption. However, some dairy products, particularly those with added sugars, can have a higher GI. Understanding which dairy products fall into this category and how they affect blood sugar levels is essential for seniors managing diabetes or looking to maintain stable energy levels.

Characteristics of High GI Dairy Products

High GI dairy products typically contain added sugars, which increase their glycemic index. These added sugars lead to faster digestion and absorption of carbohydrates, resulting in rapid spikes in blood glucose levels.

Examples of High GI Dairy Products

1. **Flavored Yogurt:**
   - **GI Score:** Approximately 50-70 (varies based on sugar content)
   - **Nutritional Benefits:** Flavored yogurts can provide calcium, protein, and probiotics. However, the high sugar content diminishes these benefits and can contribute to increased blood sugar levels.
   - **Considerations:** Opt for plain yogurt and add fresh fruits or a small amount of honey to control sugar intake.
2. **Ice Cream:**
   - **GI Score:** Approximately 60-80
   - **Nutritional Benefits:** Ice cream provides calcium and some protein but is high in added sugars and fats, leading to a higher GI.

- **Considerations:** Choose low-sugar or no-added-sugar versions, or consider frozen yogurt or sorbet with lower sugar content.

3. **Sweetened Condensed Milk:**
   - **GI Score:** Approximately 60-80
   - **Nutritional Benefits:** Sweetened condensed milk is rich in calcium and vitamin D but also high in added sugars, making it a high GI dairy product.
   - **Considerations:** Use sparingly and consider diluting with regular milk to reduce sugar content.

4. **Chocolate Milk:**
   - **GI Score:** Approximately 35-45 (varies based on sugar content)
   - **Nutritional Benefits:** Chocolate milk provides calcium, protein, and vitamins A and D. However, the added sugar content increases its GI.
   - **Considerations:** Opt for low-sugar or no-added-sugar versions, or make your own by mixing unsweetened cocoa powder with milk and a natural sweetener.

5. **Flavored Milk Drinks:**
   - **GI Score:** Approximately 45-60
   - **Nutritional Benefits:** Flavored milk drinks offer calcium, protein, and vitamins but often contain high levels of added sugars, raising their GI.
   - **Considerations:** Choose unsweetened versions or flavor plain milk with natural ingredients like vanilla extract or a small amount of fruit.

Managing High GI Dairy Products in the Diet

While high GI dairy products can cause rapid increases in blood sugar levels, they can still be enjoyed in moderation and with mindful choices. Here are some strategies for managing high GI dairy products:

1. **Opt for Low-Sugar Alternatives:**
   - Choose dairy products with no added sugars or those labeled as low-sugar or unsweetened.

- *Examples:* Plain yogurt instead of flavored yogurt, unsweetened almond milk instead of chocolate milk.

2. **Add Natural Sweeteners:**
   - Sweeten plain dairy products with natural sweeteners like fruits, honey, or stevia to control sugar intake and lower the GI.
     - *Examples:* Add fresh berries to plain yogurt or a teaspoon of honey to plain milk.

3. **Watch Portion Sizes:**
   - Keep portion sizes small to minimize the impact on blood sugar levels.
     - *Examples:* Enjoy a small scoop of ice cream as an occasional treat rather than a large serving.

4. **Combine with Low GI Foods:**
   - Pair high GI dairy products with low GI foods to balance the overall glycemic impact of the meal.
     - *Examples:* Mix flavored yogurt with nuts and seeds or have a small serving of ice cream with a fiber-rich fruit like berries.

5. **Read Labels Carefully:**
   - Pay attention to nutrition labels to identify hidden sugars and choose products with lower sugar content.
     - *Examples:* Check for added sugars in flavored yogurts and milk drinks.

6. **Make Homemade Versions:**
   - Prepare homemade versions of high GI dairy products to control the ingredients and reduce sugar content.
     - *Examples:* Make homemade chocolate milk with unsweetened cocoa powder and a natural sweetener.

Example Meal Combinations

1. **Breakfast:**
   - **Plain Yogurt with Fresh Fruit:** Combine plain yogurt with fresh fruit like strawberries or blueberries for a nutrient-rich and lower GI breakfast option.
2. **Snack:**
   - **Homemade Chocolate Milk:** Mix unsweetened cocoa powder with plain milk and a small amount of stevia or honey for a lower GI chocolate milk.
3. **Dessert:**
   - **Frozen Yogurt with Nuts:** Enjoy a small serving of low-sugar frozen yogurt topped with a handful of nuts for added protein and fiber.
4. **Beverage:**
   - **Vanilla Almond Milk:** Flavor unsweetened almond milk with a few drops of vanilla extract for a tasty and low-GI beverage.

High GI dairy products, such as flavored yogurt, ice cream, sweetened condensed milk, chocolate milk, and flavored milk drinks, contain added sugars that can lead to rapid spikes in blood sugar levels. While these products can be enjoyed occasionally, it is important for seniors to choose low-sugar alternatives, monitor portion sizes, and combine them with low GI foods to manage their glycemic impact. By making mindful choices and opting for healthier versions, seniors can still enjoy dairy products while maintaining stable blood sugar levels and overall health.

4.4.2 Medium GI Dairy Products

Medium glycemic index (GI) dairy products have a GI score ranging from 56 to 69. These dairy products have a moderate impact on blood sugar levels, providing a balance between rapid energy release and sustained energy. For seniors, incorporating medium GI dairy products into the diet can offer nutritional benefits while supporting stable blood sugar levels.

Characteristics of Medium GI Dairy Products

Medium GI dairy products typically contain moderate amounts of naturally occurring sugars like lactose and may have some added sugars. They are a good source of essential nutrients, including calcium, vitamin D, and protein, which are crucial for maintaining bone health and overall well-being in seniors.

Examples of Medium GI Dairy Products

1. **Reduced-Fat Milk:**
    - **GI Score:** Approximately 34-41
    - **Nutritional Benefits:** Reduced-fat milk provides calcium, vitamin D, protein, and essential fats while being lower in fat compared to whole milk. This balance supports bone health and cardiovascular health.
    - **Considerations:** Suitable for those looking to reduce fat intake without compromising on essential nutrients.
2. **Fruit-Flavored Yogurt (without added sugars):**
    - **GI Score:** Approximately 33-39
    - **Nutritional Benefits:** Fruit-flavored yogurt provides calcium, protein, and probiotics. When no added sugars are present, the natural fruit sugars contribute to a moderate GI.
    - **Considerations:** Choose brands that use natural fruit purees and avoid those with added sugars or artificial sweeteners.

3. **Soy Milk:**
   - **GI Score:** Approximately 34-44
   - **Nutritional Benefits:** Soy milk is rich in protein, calcium (if fortified), and isoflavones, which may support heart health. It is also lactose-free, making it suitable for those with lactose intolerance.
   - **Considerations:** Opt for unsweetened versions to keep the GI moderate and avoid unnecessary sugar intake.

4. **Lactose-Free Milk:**
   - **GI Score:** Approximately 45-48
   - **Nutritional Benefits:** Lactose-free milk offers the same benefits as regular milk, such as calcium and vitamin D, but is suitable for individuals with lactose intolerance. The lactose is broken down into simpler sugars, slightly raising the GI.
   - **Considerations:** Suitable for those who need to avoid lactose but still want to enjoy the benefits of milk.

5. **Goat Milk:**
   - **GI Score:** Approximately 37
   - **Nutritional Benefits:** Goat milk is rich in calcium, vitamin D, and protein, and may be easier to digest for some people compared to cow's milk. It also contains medium-chain fatty acids that can be beneficial for health.
   - **Considerations:** Goat milk has a slightly tangy taste and can be used in place of cow's milk in various recipes.

Managing Medium GI Dairy Products in the Diet

Medium GI dairy products can be a healthy part of a balanced diet for seniors. Here are some tips for incorporating them effectively:

1. **Choose Unsweetened Versions:**
   - Select unsweetened or naturally flavored dairy products to keep the GI moderate and avoid added sugars.

- *Examples:* Unsweetened soy milk or fruit-flavored yogurt without added sugars.

2. **Monitor Portion Sizes:**
   - Keep portion sizes moderate to manage the glycemic impact while still benefiting from the nutrients.
     - *Examples:* A small glass of reduced-fat milk or a serving of yogurt.

3. **Pair with Low GI Foods:**
   - Combine medium GI dairy products with low GI foods to balance the overall glycemic impact of meals.
     - *Examples:* Pair yogurt with nuts and seeds or add soy milk to a smoothie with low GI fruits.

4. **Incorporate into Balanced Meals:**
   - Include medium GI dairy products as part of a balanced meal that includes proteins, healthy fats, and fiber.
     - *Examples:* Use lactose-free milk in oatmeal or add goat milk to a whole grain cereal.

5. **Read Labels Carefully:**
   - Check nutrition labels to ensure that medium GI dairy products do not contain hidden sugars or additives.
     - *Examples:* Look for plain or naturally flavored options without added sugars.

Example Meal Combinations

1. **Breakfast:**
   - **Oatmeal with Soy Milk:** Cook oats with unsweetened soy milk and top with fresh berries and a sprinkle of chia seeds for a nutritious and balanced breakfast.

2. **Snack:**
   - **Fruit-Flavored Yogurt with Nuts:** Enjoy a serving of fruit-flavored yogurt without added sugars, topped with a handful of nuts for added protein and healthy fats.
3. **Lunch:**
   - **Smoothie with Reduced-Fat Milk:** Blend reduced-fat milk with spinach, banana, and a spoonful of almond butter for a nutrient-dense smoothie.
4. **Dinner:**
   - **Goat Cheese Salad:** Create a salad with mixed greens, cherry tomatoes, cucumber, and a small amount of goat cheese, drizzled with olive oil and balsamic vinegar.
5. **Beverage:**
   - **Lactose-Free Milk with Cocoa:** Mix lactose-free milk with unsweetened cocoa powder and a dash of cinnamon for a warm and comforting beverage.

Medium GI dairy products, such as reduced-fat milk, fruit-flavored yogurt (without added sugars), soy milk, lactose-free milk, and goat milk, offer essential nutrients that are crucial for seniors' health. These products provide a balance between quick energy release and sustained energy, supporting stable blood sugar levels and overall well-being. By choosing unsweetened versions, monitoring portion sizes, and pairing them with low GI foods, seniors can effectively incorporate medium GI dairy products into their diet to enjoy their nutritional benefits while maintaining glycemic control.

4.4.3 Low GI Dairy Products

Low glycemic index (GI) dairy products have a GI score of 55 or below, meaning they have a minimal impact on blood sugar levels. These dairy products digest slowly, providing a steady release of glucose into the bloodstream. For seniors, including low GI dairy products in their diet can support stable blood sugar levels, improve satiety, and contribute to overall health.

Characteristics of Low GI Dairy Products

Low GI dairy products are typically rich in protein and healthy fats, which slow down the digestion and absorption of carbohydrates. They also provide essential nutrients like calcium, vitamin D, and probiotics, which are beneficial for bone health, immune function, and digestion.

Examples of Low GI Dairy Products

1. **Plain Greek Yogurt:**
   - **GI Score:** Approximately 11-15
   - **Nutritional Benefits:** Greek yogurt is high in protein, calcium, and probiotics. The high protein content helps with muscle maintenance and repair, while probiotics support gut health.
   - **Considerations:** Opt for plain, unsweetened versions to avoid added sugars and keep the GI low.
2. **Whole Milk:**
   - **GI Score:** Approximately 31
   - **Nutritional Benefits:** Whole milk provides calcium, vitamin D, and healthy fats. The fat content helps slow the absorption of carbohydrates, contributing to a lower GI.
   - **Considerations:** Whole milk can be included in moderation as part of a balanced diet.

3. **Cheese:**
    - **GI Score:** Approximately 0-2
    - **Nutritional Benefits:** Cheese is rich in protein, calcium, and healthy fats. It also contains vitamins A and B12, which support vision and nervous system health.
    - **Considerations:** Different types of cheese have different nutrient profiles, but most are low in carbohydrates, making them low GI.
4. **Cottage Cheese:**
    - **GI Score:** Approximately 10
    - **Nutritional Benefits:** Cottage cheese is a good source of protein and calcium, with a lower fat content compared to other cheeses. It also provides B vitamins and phosphorus.
    - **Considerations:** Choose low-sodium versions to manage blood pressure.
5. **Kefir:**
    - **GI Score:** Approximately 46
    - **Nutritional Benefits:** Kefir is a fermented dairy product rich in probiotics, which support gut health and immunity. It also provides protein, calcium, and vitamin D.
    - **Considerations:** Opt for plain kefir without added sugars to keep the GI low.
6. **Butter and Cream:**
    - **GI Score:** Approximately 0
    - **Nutritional Benefits:** Butter and cream are primarily composed of fats with minimal carbohydrates, contributing to a low GI. They provide fat-soluble vitamins A, D, E, and K.
    - **Considerations:** Use in moderation due to their high fat content.

Managing Low GI Dairy Products in the Diet

Low GI dairy products can be easily incorporated into a balanced diet for seniors. Here are some tips for maximizing their benefits:

1. **Incorporate into Meals and Snacks:**
   - Use low GI dairy products in a variety of meals and snacks to ensure a steady intake of essential nutrients.
     - *Examples:* Add Greek yogurt to smoothies, include cheese in salads, or use cottage cheese as a topping for whole grain toast.

2. **Pair with High Fiber Foods:**
   - Combining low GI dairy products with high fiber foods can further stabilize blood sugar levels and enhance satiety.
     - *Examples:* Mix Greek yogurt with chia seeds and berries, or have whole milk with a high-fiber cereal.

3. **Use as a Protein Source:**
   - Low GI dairy products can serve as an excellent source of protein, supporting muscle maintenance and overall health.
     - *Examples:* Enjoy cottage cheese with fruit or add cheese to an omelet.

4. **Enjoy Fermented Options:**
   - Fermented dairy products like kefir provide probiotics that support gut health and can be beneficial for overall well-being.
     - *Examples:* Drink plain kefir as a beverage or use it as a base for smoothies.

5. **Monitor Portion Sizes:**
   - While low GI dairy products are beneficial, it's important to keep portion sizes moderate to manage overall caloric intake.
     - *Examples:* Enjoy a small serving of cheese with vegetables or a moderate portion of Greek yogurt.

Example Meal Combinations

1. **Breakfast:**
   - **Greek Yogurt Parfait:** Layer plain Greek yogurt with fresh berries, a sprinkle of nuts, and a drizzle of honey for a nutritious and balanced breakfast.
2. **Snack:**
   - **Cheese and Apple Slices:** Pair slices of cheese with apple slices for a satisfying and low GI snack.
3. **Lunch:**
   - **Cottage Cheese and Veggies:** Serve cottage cheese with a side of sliced cucumbers, cherry tomatoes, and whole grain crackers.
4. **Dinner:**
   - **Kefir Smoothie:** Blend plain kefir with spinach, avocado, and a small banana for a nutrient-dense and low GI smoothie.
5. **Dessert:**
   - **Berries with Cream:** Top a bowl of mixed berries with a dollop of whipped cream for a delicious and low GI dessert.

Low GI dairy products, such as plain Greek yogurt, whole milk, cheese, cottage cheese, kefir, and butter, offer numerous health benefits for seniors. These products are rich in protein, calcium, healthy fats, and probiotics, contributing to stable blood sugar levels, improved satiety, and overall well-being. By incorporating a variety of low GI dairy products into meals and pairing them with high fiber foods, seniors can enjoy their nutritional advantages while maintaining stable blood sugar levels and promoting long-term health.

4.5 Proteins

4.5.1 High GI Protein Sources

High glycemic index (GI) protein sources are less common because proteins generally have a minimal impact on blood sugar levels. However, certain protein-rich foods can have a high GI if they are processed or contain added sugars. Understanding these high GI protein sources is essential for seniors managing blood sugar levels, as these foods can cause rapid spikes in glucose.

Characteristics of High GI Protein Sources

High GI protein sources typically contain carbohydrates in addition to protein. These carbohydrates, often in the form of sugars or starches, lead to a higher GI score. These foods may be convenient and tasty but can undermine efforts to maintain stable blood sugar levels.

Examples of High GI Protein Sources

1. **Protein Bars:**
   - **GI Score:** Approximately 60-80 (varies based on ingredients)
   - **Nutritional Benefits:** Protein bars often provide a quick and convenient source of protein. They can also contain vitamins, minerals, and fiber.
   - **Considerations:** Many protein bars are high in added sugars and refined carbohydrates, increasing their GI. It's important to read labels and choose bars with minimal added sugars and higher fiber content.
2. **Sweetened Protein Shakes:**
   - **GI Score:** Approximately 50-70 (varies based on sugar content)
   - **Nutritional Benefits:** Protein shakes can be a quick source of protein, vitamins, and minerals, especially for those with limited time or appetite.

- **Considerations:** Many commercial protein shakes contain added sugars or high-GI carbohydrate fillers. Opt for unsweetened or naturally sweetened options.

3. **Marinated Meats with Sugary Sauces:**
   - **GI Score:** Approximately 55-75 (varies based on sauce ingredients)
   - **Nutritional Benefits:** Marinated meats provide high-quality protein and essential nutrients like iron and B vitamins.
   - **Considerations:** Sauces that contain high amounts of sugar, such as barbecue or teriyaki sauces, can increase the GI of the meal. Choose marinades with low or no added sugars, or make your own using herbs and spices.

4. **Breaded and Fried Meats:**
   - **GI Score:** Approximately 70-85 (due to breading and frying process)
   - **Nutritional Benefits:** Breaded and fried meats offer protein but often come with unhealthy fats and refined carbohydrates.
   - **Considerations:** The breading and frying process adds refined carbohydrates and unhealthy fats, significantly raising the GI. Opt for grilled, baked, or steamed protein sources instead.

Managing High GI Protein Sources in the Diet

While high GI protein sources can be convenient and tasty, it is important to manage their intake to avoid rapid blood sugar spikes. Here are some strategies:

1. **Choose Low-Sugar Options:**
   - Select protein bars and shakes with minimal added sugars and higher fiber content.
     - *Examples:* Look for bars with whole food ingredients like nuts and seeds, and shakes sweetened with natural alternatives like stevia.
2. **Make Your Own Protein Snacks:**
   - Prepare homemade protein bars and shakes to control ingredients and reduce added sugars.

- ■ *Examples:* Blend protein powder with unsweetened almond milk, spinach, and a small banana for a healthy shake.

3. **Opt for Natural Protein Sources:**
   - ○ Choose whole, unprocessed protein sources to maintain a low GI diet.
     - ■ *Examples:* Grilled chicken, turkey, or fish instead of breaded and fried versions.

4. **Read Labels Carefully:**
   - ○ Check ingredient lists and nutrition labels for added sugars and high-GI carbohydrates.
     - ■ *Examples:* Avoid protein bars and shakes with high fructose corn syrup or other refined sugars.

5. **Use Low-GI Marinades:**
   - ○ Marinate meats with herbs, spices, and low-sugar ingredients.
     - ■ *Examples:* Use olive oil, lemon juice, garlic, and rosemary for a flavorful, low-GI marinade.

Example Meal Combinations

1. **Breakfast:**
   - ○ **Homemade Protein Shake:** Blend protein powder with unsweetened almond milk, spinach, and a handful of berries for a nutrient-dense, low-GI shake.

2. **Snack:**
   - ○ **Low-Sugar Protein Bar:** Choose a protein bar made with whole food ingredients and minimal added sugars, such as nuts, seeds, and dates.

3. **Lunch:**
   - ○ **Grilled Chicken Salad:** Top a mixed greens salad with grilled chicken breast, avocado, and a low-sugar vinaigrette.

4. **Dinner:**
   - **Herb-Marinated Fish:** Marinate fish fillets with olive oil, lemon juice, garlic, and fresh herbs, then grill or bake for a flavorful and low-GI protein source.

5. **Dessert:**
   - **Greek Yogurt with Nuts:** Enjoy a serving of plain Greek yogurt topped with a handful of nuts and a drizzle of honey for a balanced, low-GI treat.

High GI protein sources, such as protein bars, sweetened protein shakes, marinated meats with sugary sauces, and breaded and fried meats, can cause rapid spikes in blood sugar levels. For seniors managing diabetes or looking to maintain stable energy levels, it is important to choose low-sugar options, prepare homemade snacks, opt for natural protein sources, read labels carefully, and use low-GI marinades. By making mindful choices, seniors can still enjoy protein-rich foods while supporting their overall health and well-being.

4.5.2 Medium GI Protein Sources

Medium glycemic index (GI) protein sources have a GI score ranging from 56 to 69. These foods provide a balanced release of glucose into the bloodstream, offering both quick energy and sustained satiety. For seniors, medium GI protein sources can be a healthy part of the diet, helping to maintain stable blood sugar levels and providing essential nutrients for overall health.

Characteristics of Medium GI Protein Sources

Medium GI protein sources often contain moderate amounts of carbohydrates alongside protein. These carbohydrates can be naturally occurring or added during processing. While they raise blood sugar levels moderately, they also offer nutritional benefits that support a balanced diet.

Examples of Medium GI Protein Sources

1. **Lentils:**
   - **GI Score:** Approximately 26-42 (depends on the type)
   - **Nutritional Benefits:** Lentils are high in protein, fiber, iron, and folate. They are a plant-based protein source that supports heart health and digestive health.
   - **Considerations:** Pair lentils with whole grains to make a complete protein.
2. **Chickpeas (Garbanzo Beans):**
   - **GI Score:** Approximately 28-42
   - **Nutritional Benefits:** Chickpeas provide protein, fiber, iron, and magnesium. They help maintain satiety and support blood sugar control.
   - **Considerations:** Use in salads, stews, or as a base for hummus.
3. **Quinoa:**
   - **GI Score:** Approximately 53

- **Nutritional Benefits:** Quinoa is a complete protein, containing all nine essential amino acids. It is also high in fiber, magnesium, and antioxidants.
    - **Considerations:** Use quinoa as a base for salads or as a side dish.
4. **Couscous:**
    - **GI Score:** Approximately 65
    - **Nutritional Benefits:** Couscous is a source of protein and selenium. It is quick to cook and can be a versatile addition to meals.
    - **Considerations:** Opt for whole wheat couscous for added fiber and nutrients.
5. **Edamame (Young Soybeans):**
    - **GI Score:** Approximately 18
    - **Nutritional Benefits:** Edamame is rich in protein, fiber, iron, and calcium. It is a convenient and nutritious snack or addition to meals.
    - **Considerations:** Enjoy steamed or added to salads and stir-fries.

Managing Medium GI Protein Sources in the Diet

Medium GI protein sources can be effectively integrated into a balanced diet for seniors. Here are some strategies:

1. **Combine with Low GI Foods:**
    - Pair medium GI protein sources with low GI foods to balance the overall glycemic impact of meals.
        - *Examples:* Mix quinoa with vegetables or serve chickpeas with leafy greens.
2. **Monitor Portion Sizes:**
    - Keep portion sizes moderate to manage blood sugar levels while enjoying the nutritional benefits.
        - *Examples:* A serving of lentils or quinoa as part of a meal.
3. **Include a Variety of Protein Sources:**
    - Incorporate a variety of medium GI protein sources to ensure a range of nutrients and avoid dietary monotony.

- *Examples:* Alternate between lentils, chickpeas, quinoa, and edamame in meal planning.

4. **Prepare Balanced Meals:**
   - Create meals that include medium GI protein sources alongside healthy fats, fiber, and low GI carbohydrates.
     - *Examples:* A quinoa salad with avocado and mixed greens or a lentil stew with vegetables.

5. **Cook from Scratch:**
   - Preparing meals from scratch allows for better control over ingredients and GI levels.
     - *Examples:* Homemade hummus with chickpeas and olive oil or a quinoa bowl with fresh vegetables.

Example Meal Combinations

1. **Breakfast:**
   - **Quinoa Breakfast Bowl:** Cook quinoa and mix with almond milk, fresh berries, and a sprinkle of nuts for a protein-packed breakfast.
2. **Snack:**
   - **Edamame:** Enjoy a bowl of steamed edamame with a pinch of sea salt for a nutritious and satisfying snack.
3. **Lunch:**
   - **Chickpea Salad:** Combine chickpeas with chopped vegetables, olive oil, and lemon juice for a refreshing and balanced salad.
4. **Dinner:**
   - **Lentil Stew:** Prepare a hearty lentil stew with carrots, celery, onions, and tomatoes, seasoned with herbs and spices.
5. **Dessert:**
   - **Quinoa Pudding:** Cook quinoa with coconut milk, a dash of cinnamon, and a touch of honey for a healthy dessert option.

Medium GI protein sources, such as lentils, chickpeas, quinoa, couscous, and edamame, offer a balance of quick and sustained energy release, helping to maintain stable blood sugar levels. These foods provide essential nutrients that support overall health and well-being. By combining them with low GI foods, monitoring portion sizes, including a variety of protein sources, preparing balanced meals, and cooking from scratch, seniors can effectively incorporate medium GI protein sources into their diet to enjoy their nutritional benefits and support long-term health.

4.5.3 Low GI Protein Sources

Low glycemic index (GI) protein sources have a GI score of 55 or below, meaning they have a minimal impact on blood sugar levels. These foods provide a steady release of energy, supporting stable blood sugar levels, satiety, and overall health. For seniors, incorporating low GI protein sources into their diet can help manage blood sugar levels, support muscle maintenance, and promote overall well-being.

Characteristics of Low GI Protein Sources

Low GI protein sources are generally high in protein and low in carbohydrates, which helps to slow the digestion and absorption of nutrients, leading to a more gradual release of glucose into the bloodstream. They are essential for muscle repair and maintenance, immune function, and various other physiological processes.

Examples of Low GI Protein Sources

1. **Lean Meats:**
   - **GI Score:** Approximately 0 (no carbohydrates)
   - **Nutritional Benefits:** Lean meats such as chicken breast, turkey, and lean cuts of beef and pork are rich in high-quality protein, iron, B vitamins, and essential amino acids.
   - **Considerations:** Choose lean cuts to minimize saturated fat intake and opt for grilling, baking, or steaming instead of frying.
2. **Fish and Seafood:**
   - **GI Score:** Approximately 0 (no carbohydrates)
   - **Nutritional Benefits:** Fish and seafood, such as salmon, tuna, cod, shrimp, and scallops, are excellent sources of protein, omega-3 fatty acids, iodine, and selenium.
   - **Considerations:** Include fatty fish like salmon and mackerel in your diet to benefit from their high omega-3 content, which supports heart health.

3. **Eggs:**
    - **GI Score:** Approximately 0 (no carbohydrates)
    - **Nutritional Benefits:** Eggs are a complete protein source, providing all nine essential amino acids. They also contain vitamins A, D, E, and B12, as well as choline, which is important for brain health.
    - **Considerations:** Enjoy eggs in moderation due to their cholesterol content, and consider boiling, poaching, or scrambling them for a healthy meal.

4. **Tofu and Tempeh:**
    - **GI Score:** Approximately 15-20
    - **Nutritional Benefits:** Tofu and tempeh are plant-based protein sources made from soybeans. They provide protein, iron, calcium, and other minerals, and are low in carbohydrates.
    - **Considerations:** Tofu is versatile and can be used in a variety of dishes, while tempeh has a firmer texture and is rich in probiotics.

5. **Nuts and Seeds:**
    - **GI Score:** Approximately 0-20 (varies by type)
    - **Nutritional Benefits:** Nuts and seeds, such as almonds, walnuts, chia seeds, and flaxseeds, are rich in protein, healthy fats, fiber, vitamins, and minerals.
    - **Considerations:** Consume in moderation due to their high calorie content, and choose unsalted and raw or lightly roasted varieties.

6. **Greek Yogurt:**
    - **GI Score:** Approximately 11-15
    - **Nutritional Benefits:** Greek yogurt is high in protein and probiotics, which support gut health. It also provides calcium, vitamin D, and potassium.
    - **Considerations:** Opt for plain, unsweetened Greek yogurt to keep the GI low and add fresh fruit or nuts for flavor.

Managing Low GI Protein Sources in the Diet

Low GI protein sources can be easily incorporated into a balanced diet for seniors. Here are some strategies:

1. **Combine with Low GI Carbohydrates:**
   - Pair low GI protein sources with low GI carbohydrates to create balanced meals that support stable blood sugar levels.
     - *Examples:* Serve grilled chicken with quinoa and vegetables, or enjoy salmon with a side of lentils and spinach.

2. **Incorporate Healthy Fats:**
   - Include healthy fats in meals to further slow digestion and enhance satiety.
     - *Examples:* Add avocado slices to an egg breakfast or drizzle olive oil on a tofu and vegetable stir-fry.

3. **Prepare Balanced Meals:**
   - Create meals that include a variety of food groups, ensuring adequate protein, healthy fats, fiber, and micronutrients.
     - *Examples:* A mixed greens salad with grilled shrimp, nuts, and a lemon vinaigrette, or a bowl of Greek yogurt topped with chia seeds and berries.

4. **Use Diverse Cooking Methods:**
   - Experiment with different cooking methods to keep meals interesting and nutritious.
     - *Examples:* Bake, grill, or steam fish and seafood, or stir-fry tofu with vegetables.

5. **Monitor Portion Sizes:**
   - Keep portion sizes appropriate to manage overall caloric intake while still benefiting from the nutrients in low GI protein sources.
     - *Examples:* A serving of lean meat about the size of a deck of cards, or a handful of nuts as a snack.

Example Meal Combinations

1. **Breakfast:**
   - **Scrambled Eggs with Spinach:** Scramble eggs with fresh spinach and serve with a side of avocado for a protein-rich and low GI breakfast.
2. **Snack:**
   - **Greek Yogurt with Berries:** Enjoy a bowl of plain Greek yogurt topped with fresh berries and a sprinkle of flaxseeds.
3. **Lunch:**
   - **Grilled Chicken Salad:** Combine mixed greens, grilled chicken breast, cherry tomatoes, cucumbers, and a lemon vinaigrette for a nutritious and balanced salad.
4. **Dinner:**
   - **Baked Salmon with Quinoa:** Serve baked salmon with a side of quinoa and steamed broccoli for a complete and satisfying meal.
5. **Dessert:**
   - **Chia Seed Pudding:** Make chia seed pudding with unsweetened almond milk and top with a few slices of fresh fruit.

Low GI protein sources, such as lean meats, fish and seafood, eggs, tofu, tempeh, nuts, seeds, and Greek yogurt, offer numerous health benefits for seniors. These foods support stable blood sugar levels, muscle maintenance, and overall well-being. By combining them with low GI carbohydrates, incorporating healthy fats, preparing balanced meals, using diverse cooking methods, and monitoring portion sizes, seniors can effectively integrate low GI protein sources into their diet to enjoy their nutritional advantages and support long-term health.

4.6 Snacks and Sweets

4.6.1 High GI Snacks

High glycemic index (GI) snacks have a GI score of 70 or above, leading to a rapid increase in blood sugar levels. These snacks typically cause a quick spike in glucose followed by a subsequent drop, which can affect energy levels and appetite. For seniors, managing high GI snacks is important to maintain stable blood sugar levels and overall health.

Characteristics of High GI Snacks

High GI snacks are often high in refined carbohydrates and sugars. These snacks can be convenient and tasty but may lack nutritional value. Understanding and managing the consumption of high GI snacks is crucial for maintaining balanced energy levels and preventing blood sugar spikes.

Examples of High GI Snacks

1. **Sugary Granola Bars:**
   - **GI Score:** Approximately 70-80 (varies based on ingredients)
   - **Nutritional Benefits:** Granola bars can provide a quick source of energy and may contain vitamins and minerals.
   - **Considerations:** Many commercially available granola bars are high in added sugars and refined carbohydrates, leading to a high GI. Opt for bars with low sugar content and high fiber.
2. **Potato Chips:**
   - **GI Score:** Approximately 70-80
   - **Nutritional Benefits:** Potato chips offer a crunchy and satisfying snack, providing some vitamins and minerals.

- **Considerations:** The high GI is due to the processing and frying of potatoes, which increases the glycemic load. Consider baked or air-fried alternatives and watch portion sizes.

3. **White Bread Sandwiches:**
   - **GI Score:** Approximately 70-80 (depends on filling and bread type)
   - **Nutritional Benefits:** White bread sandwiches can be a convenient and quick snack option.
   - **Considerations:** White bread is made from refined flour, which contributes to a high GI. Choose whole grain or high-fiber breads to lower the GI.

4. **Candy and Chocolate Bars:**
   - **GI Score:** Approximately 70-90 (varies by type)
   - **Nutritional Benefits:** Candy and chocolate bars can provide quick energy and may contain some antioxidants (in dark chocolate).
   - **Considerations:** These snacks are high in sugar and fat, leading to a high GI. Opt for dark chocolate with lower sugar content and consume in moderation.

5. **Sweetened Yogurt:**
   - **GI Score:** Approximately 60-80 (depends on sugar content)
   - **Nutritional Benefits:** Sweetened yogurt can provide protein and calcium.
   - **Considerations:** Many flavored yogurts contain added sugars that increase their GI. Choose plain, unsweetened yogurt and add fresh fruit or nuts for flavor.

6. **Soft Drinks and Fruit Juices:**
   - **GI Score:** Approximately 70-80 (varies by type)
   - **Nutritional Benefits:** These beverages offer a quick source of hydration and energy.

- ○ **Considerations:** Soft drinks and fruit juices are high in sugar, which leads to a high GI. Opt for water, herbal teas, or diluted fruit juices to manage sugar intake.

Managing High GI Snacks in the Diet

While high GI snacks can be tempting, it's important to manage their consumption to avoid rapid blood sugar spikes. Here are some strategies:

1. **Limit Portion Sizes:**
   - ○ Keep portions small to minimize the impact on blood sugar levels.
     - ■ *Examples:* Enjoy a small piece of chocolate or a few potato chips as a treat.

2. **Pair with Low GI Foods:**
   - ○ Combine high GI snacks with low GI foods to balance their effect on blood sugar.
     - ■ *Examples:* Pair a granola bar with a handful of nuts or a piece of fruit.

3. **Choose Nutrient-Dense Options:**
   - ○ Opt for snacks that provide additional nutrients beyond just carbohydrates and sugars.
     - ■ *Examples:* Select granola bars with nuts and seeds or dark chocolate with a higher cocoa content.

4. **Prepare Homemade Snacks:**
   - ○ Make snacks at home to control ingredients and avoid excessive sugars and refined carbohydrates.
     - ■ *Examples:* Bake whole grain crackers or prepare homemade trail mix with nuts and dried fruit.

5. **Read Labels Carefully:**
   - ○ Check nutrition labels for sugar content and overall GI impact.
     - ■ *Examples:* Avoid snacks with high fructose corn syrup or excessive added sugars.

Example Snack Combinations

1. **Breakfast:**
   - **Greek Yogurt with Fresh Berries:** Choose plain Greek yogurt and add a handful of fresh berries for a balanced snack.
2. **Snack:**
   - **Nuts and a Small Piece of Dark Chocolate:** Enjoy a small piece of dark chocolate with a handful of almonds or walnuts.
3. **Lunch:**
   - **Whole Grain Crackers with Hummus:** Pair whole grain crackers with a serving of hummus for a satisfying and balanced snack.
4. **Dinner:**
   - **Baked Sweet Potato Fries:** Make baked sweet potato fries with a sprinkle of paprika for a lower GI alternative to regular potato chips.
5. **Dessert:**
   - **Chia Seed Pudding:** Prepare chia seed pudding with unsweetened almond milk and a touch of honey for a low GI dessert.

High GI snacks, such as sugary granola bars, potato chips, white bread sandwiches, candy, sweetened yogurt, and soft drinks, can lead to rapid blood sugar spikes and fluctuating energy levels. For seniors managing blood sugar levels, it's important to limit high GI snacks, choose nutrient-dense options, pair them with low GI foods, and prepare snacks at home when possible. By making mindful choices and managing portion sizes, seniors can enjoy their snacks while maintaining stable blood sugar levels and overall health.

4.6.2 Medium GI Snacks

Medium glycemic index (GI) snacks have a GI score ranging from 56 to 69. These snacks provide a moderate increase in blood sugar levels, offering a balanced energy boost without causing rapid spikes. For seniors, medium GI snacks can be a good choice for maintaining steady energy levels and managing hunger while providing essential nutrients.

Characteristics of Medium GI Snacks

Medium GI snacks typically contain moderate amounts of carbohydrates that are digested and absorbed at a moderate rate. They can offer a combination of protein, fiber, and healthy fats, which help stabilize blood sugar levels and keep you satisfied longer.

Examples of Medium GI Snacks

1. **Whole Grain Crackers:**
   - **GI Score:** Approximately 60-65
   - **Nutritional Benefits:** Whole grain crackers are a source of complex carbohydrates and fiber. They can provide sustained energy and help with digestive health.
   - **Considerations:** Choose crackers with minimal added sugars and healthy fats. Pair with a protein source for a balanced snack.
2. **Oatmeal:**
   - **GI Score:** Approximately 55-65 (depends on type)
   - **Nutritional Benefits:** Oatmeal is rich in fiber, particularly beta-glucan, which helps lower cholesterol and support heart health. It also provides steady energy.
   - **Considerations:** Opt for steel-cut or old-fashioned oats over instant oatmeal, which often has added sugars.

3. **Apple Slices with Peanut Butter:**
   - **GI Score:** Approximately 55-65
   - **Nutritional Benefits:** Apples provide fiber and vitamins, while peanut butter adds protein and healthy fats. This combination helps stabilize blood sugar levels and keeps you full.
   - **Considerations:** Use natural peanut butter without added sugars or hydrogenated fats. Watch portion sizes to manage calorie intake.

4. **Hummus with Carrot Sticks:**
   - **GI Score:** Approximately 60-65
   - **Nutritional Benefits:** Hummus is a good source of protein and fiber from chickpeas, and carrots provide vitamins and additional fiber. This snack supports steady energy and digestive health.
   - **Considerations:** Choose hummus made from whole, natural ingredients, and avoid varieties with added sugars.

5. **Greek Yogurt with Honey and Nuts:**
   - **GI Score:** Approximately 55-65 (depends on amount of honey)
   - **Nutritional Benefits:** Greek yogurt provides protein and probiotics, while nuts offer healthy fats and additional protein. Honey adds a touch of natural sweetness.
   - **Considerations:** Use raw honey and watch portion sizes. Opt for plain Greek yogurt to avoid added sugars.

6. **Popcorn (Air-Popped):**
   - **GI Score:** Approximately 55-60
   - **Nutritional Benefits:** Air-popped popcorn is high in fiber and low in calories, making it a filling and satisfying snack. It also provides a small amount of protein.
   - **Considerations:** Avoid adding too much salt or butter. Season with herbs or spices for flavor without increasing the GI.

Managing Medium GI Snacks in the Diet

Medium GI snacks can be incorporated into a balanced diet with some considerations to ensure they contribute to stable blood sugar levels and overall health. Here are some strategies:

1. **Pair with Low GI Foods:**
   - Combine medium GI snacks with low GI foods to balance their impact on blood sugar.
     - *Examples:* Pair oatmeal with a small amount of nuts or fruit, or enjoy whole grain crackers with a slice of cheese.

2. **Monitor Portion Sizes:**
   - Keep portion sizes in check to manage overall calorie and carbohydrate intake.
     - *Examples:* A small serving of hummus with carrot sticks or a modest bowl of oatmeal.

3. **Include Protein and Fiber:**
   - Ensure snacks contain protein and fiber to help keep you full and stabilize blood sugar levels.
     - *Examples:* Greek yogurt with nuts, or apple slices with peanut butter.

4. **Prepare Snacks at Home:**
   - Homemade snacks allow for better control over ingredients and help avoid added sugars and unhealthy fats.
     - *Examples:* Make your own oatmeal with fruit and nuts or prepare homemade hummus.

5. **Read Labels Carefully:**
   - When purchasing snacks, check labels for added sugars, sodium, and other additives.
     - *Examples:* Choose whole grain crackers without added sugars or artificial ingredients.

Example Snack Combinations

1. **Breakfast:**
   - **Oatmeal with Fresh Berries:** Cook oatmeal and top with fresh berries and a sprinkle of chia seeds for a nutritious and filling breakfast.
2. **Snack:**
   - **Apple Slices with Natural Peanut Butter:** Enjoy apple slices with a tablespoon of natural peanut butter for a satisfying and balanced snack.
3. **Lunch:**
   - **Whole Grain Crackers with Hummus:** Pair whole grain crackers with a serving of hummus and a side of sliced vegetables.
4. **Dinner:**
   - **Greek Yogurt with Nuts and Honey:** Have a serving of plain Greek yogurt topped with a handful of nuts and a drizzle of honey.
5. **Dessert:**
   - **Air-Popped Popcorn:** Enjoy a bowl of air-popped popcorn seasoned with your favorite herbs or spices.

Medium GI snacks, such as whole grain crackers, oatmeal, apple slices with peanut butter, hummus with carrot sticks, Greek yogurt with honey and nuts, and air-popped popcorn, offer a balanced increase in blood sugar levels and provide essential nutrients. By pairing them with low GI foods, monitoring portion sizes, including protein and fiber, preparing snacks at home, and reading labels carefully, seniors can enjoy these snacks while maintaining stable blood sugar levels and overall health.

4.6.3 Low GI Snacks

Low glycemic index (GI) snacks have a GI score of 55 or below, meaning they have a minimal impact on blood sugar levels. These snacks provide a steady and gradual release of glucose into the bloodstream, helping to maintain stable energy levels and prevent rapid spikes and crashes in blood sugar. For seniors, incorporating low GI snacks into their diet is beneficial for overall health and blood sugar management.

Characteristics of Low GI Snacks

Low GI snacks typically contain complex carbohydrates, fiber, protein, and healthy fats, which help slow digestion and promote sustained energy. These snacks are often nutrient-dense, providing essential vitamins, minerals, and other beneficial compounds.

Examples of Low GI Snacks

1. **Nuts and Seeds:**
   - **GI Score:** Approximately 0-20 (varies by type)
   - **Nutritional Benefits:** Nuts and seeds are rich in protein, healthy fats, fiber, vitamins, and minerals. They help stabilize blood sugar levels and provide sustained satiety.
   - **Considerations:** Opt for unsalted and raw or lightly roasted varieties. Examples include almonds, walnuts, chia seeds, and flaxseeds.
2. **Vegetable Sticks with Hummus:**
   - **GI Score:** Approximately 25-35
   - **Nutritional Benefits:** Fresh vegetable sticks, such as carrots, celery, and bell peppers, provide fiber, vitamins, and minerals. Hummus adds protein and healthy fats from chickpeas.
   - **Considerations:** Choose hummus made from whole ingredients and avoid varieties with added sugars.
3. **Greek Yogurt (Plain, Unsweetened):**
   - **GI Score:** Approximately 11-15

- **Nutritional Benefits:** Plain Greek yogurt is high in protein and probiotics, supporting gut health. It also provides calcium and potassium.
  - **Considerations:** Add fresh fruit or a small amount of nuts for added flavor and nutrition without significantly increasing the GI.

4. **Hard-Boiled Eggs:**
   - **GI Score:** Approximately 0 (no carbohydrates)
   - **Nutritional Benefits:** Hard-boiled eggs are a complete protein source and provide essential nutrients like vitamins A, D, E, and B12.
   - **Considerations:** Enjoy as a convenient and portable snack. Season with herbs or a sprinkle of pepper for added flavor.

5. **Edamame:**
   - **GI Score:** Approximately 18
   - **Nutritional Benefits:** Edamame (young soybeans) is a high-protein, fiber-rich snack that also provides iron and calcium. It is a satisfying and nutritious option.
   - **Considerations:** Enjoy steamed or lightly salted. Edamame can also be added to salads and other dishes.

6. **Cottage Cheese:**
   - **GI Score:** Approximately 10-15
   - **Nutritional Benefits:** Cottage cheese is high in protein and calcium. It provides a satisfying snack option and supports muscle maintenance and bone health.
   - **Considerations:** Opt for low-fat or fat-free varieties to reduce saturated fat intake. Pair with fruit or vegetables for a balanced snack.

7. **Chia Seed Pudding:**
   - **GI Score:** Approximately 30
   - **Nutritional Benefits:** Chia seeds are rich in omega-3 fatty acids, fiber, and protein. When soaked, they form a gel-like pudding that is both filling and nutritious.

    ○ **Considerations:** Prepare with unsweetened almond milk and add a touch of natural sweetener or fresh fruit.

Managing Low GI Snacks in the Diet

Incorporating low GI snacks into a balanced diet can help seniors maintain stable blood sugar levels and support overall health. Here are some strategies:

1. **Pair with Protein or Healthy Fats:**
   ○ Combine low GI snacks with protein or healthy fats to enhance satiety and nutritional value.
      ■ *Examples:* Pair vegetable sticks with hummus or nuts with Greek yogurt.
2. **Incorporate Variety:**
   ○ Include a range of low GI snacks to ensure a diverse intake of nutrients and to prevent dietary monotony.
      ■ *Examples:* Rotate between nuts, Greek yogurt, and hard-boiled eggs.
3. **Prepare Snacks at Home:**
   ○ Making snacks at home allows for better control over ingredients and helps avoid added sugars and unhealthy fats.
      ■ *Examples:* Prepare chia seed pudding or make your own hummus.
4. **Monitor Portion Sizes:**
   ○ Keep portion sizes appropriate to manage calorie and nutrient intake effectively.
      ■ *Examples:* A small handful of nuts or a serving of Greek yogurt.
5. **Include Snacks in Balanced Meals:**
   ○ Ensure that snacks contribute to the overall balance of the meal plan, complementing other meals and snacks.
      ■ *Examples:* Enjoy cottage cheese with a side of fruit or edamame as a mid-afternoon snack.

Example Snack Combinations

1. **Breakfast:**
   - **Greek Yogurt with Chia Seeds:** Mix plain Greek yogurt with chia seeds and top with a few fresh berries for a nutritious start to the day.
2. **Snack:**
   - **Nuts and Seeds Mix:** Enjoy a handful of almonds and flaxseeds for a satisfying and nutrient-dense snack.
3. **Lunch:**
   - **Vegetable Sticks with Hummus:** Pair carrot and celery sticks with a serving of hummus for a crunchy and protein-rich snack.
4. **Dinner:**
   - **Hard-Boiled Eggs:** Have a couple of hard-boiled eggs with a side of sliced avocado for a filling and protein-packed snack.
5. **Dessert:**
   - **Chia Seed Pudding:** Prepare chia seed pudding with unsweetened almond milk and a touch of vanilla extract, and enjoy it as a light dessert.

Low GI snacks, such as nuts and seeds, vegetable sticks with hummus, plain Greek yogurt, hard-boiled eggs, edamame, cottage cheese, and chia seed pudding, offer a steady release of glucose into the bloodstream, supporting stable blood sugar levels and overall health. By pairing them with protein or healthy fats, incorporating variety, preparing snacks at home, monitoring portion sizes, and including snacks in balanced meals, seniors can effectively enjoy these nutritious options while maintaining long-term health and well-being.

Chapter 5: Meal Planning and Recipes

5.1 Breakfast Ideas

1. Whole Grain Toast with Avocado and Poached Egg

Ingredients:

- 1 slice whole grain bread
- 1/2 ripe avocado
- 1 large egg
- Salt and pepper to taste
- Fresh herbs (optional, e.g., chives or parsley)

Directions:

1. **Toast Bread:** Toast the whole grain bread until golden brown.
2. **Prepare Avocado:** While the bread is toasting, mash the avocado in a small bowl. Season with a pinch of salt and pepper.
3. **Poach Egg:** Fill a small saucepan with water and bring to a gentle simmer. Crack the egg into a small bowl. Create a gentle whirlpool in the water and carefully slide the egg into the center. Poach for about 3-4 minutes until the white is set but the yolk is still runny. Remove with a slotted spoon.
4. **Assemble:** Spread the mashed avocado on the toasted bread. Top with the poached egg. Season with additional salt, pepper, and fresh herbs if desired.

Cooking and Prep Time:

- **Prep Time:** 5 minutes
- **Cooking Time:** 5-7 minutes
- **Total Time:** 10-12 minutes

Servings: 1

Nutritional Information (approximate):

- Calories: 290
- Protein: 12g
- Carbohydrates: 26g
- Fiber: 7g
- Fat: 17g
- Saturated Fat: 3g
- Sodium: 300mg

2. Greek Yogurt with Fresh Fruit and Nuts

Ingredients:

- 1 cup plain Greek yogurt
- 1/2 cup fresh berries (e.g., strawberries, blueberries, or raspberries)
- 2 tbsp chopped almonds or walnuts
- 1 tsp honey (optional)

Directions:

1. **Prepare Yogurt:** Scoop the Greek yogurt into a bowl.
2. **Add Fruit:** Wash and slice the fresh berries, then add them to the yogurt.
3. **Top with Nuts:** Sprinkle the chopped almonds or walnuts over the yogurt and berries.
4. **Sweeten (Optional):** Drizzle a teaspoon of honey over the top if desired.

Cooking and Prep Time:

- **Prep Time:** 5 minutes
- **Cooking Time:** None

- **Total Time:** 5 minutes

Servings: 1

Nutritional Information (approximate):

- Calories: 320
- Protein: 20g
- Carbohydrates: 28g
- Fiber: 5g
- Fat: 17g
- Saturated Fat: 1.5g
- Sodium: 80mg

3. Vegetable and Egg Muffins

Ingredients:

- 4 large eggs
- 1/2 cup chopped bell peppers (any color)
- 1/2 cup chopped spinach
- 1/4 cup chopped onion
- 1/4 cup shredded cheese (optional, e.g., cheddar or feta)
- Salt and pepper to taste
- Cooking spray or a small amount of oil for greasing the muffin tin

Directions:

1. **Preheat Oven:** Preheat your oven to 375°F (190°C). Grease a muffin tin or line with paper liners.
2. **Prepare Vegetables:** Chop bell peppers, spinach, and onion.

3. **Mix Ingredients:** In a bowl, whisk the eggs and season with salt and pepper. Stir in the chopped vegetables and cheese if using.
4. **Fill Muffin Tin:** Pour the egg mixture evenly into the muffin tin cups.
5. **Bake:** Bake for 20-25 minutes or until the muffins are set and slightly golden on top. A toothpick inserted into the center should come out clean.
6. **Cool and Serve:** Allow to cool slightly before removing from the tin. Serve warm or at room temperature.

Cooking and Prep Time:

- **Prep Time:** 10 minutes
- **Cooking Time:** 20-25 minutes
- **Total Time:** 30-35 minutes

Servings: 4 muffins (1 muffin per serving)

Nutritional Information (per muffin, approximate):

- Calories: 100
- Protein: 7g
- Carbohydrates: 4g
- Fiber: 1g
- Fat: 7g
- Saturated Fat: 2g
- Sodium: 200mg

5.2 Lunch Ideas

1. Quinoa Salad with Chickpeas and Vegetables

Ingredients:

- 1 cup cooked quinoa (cooled)
- 1/2 cup canned chickpeas (rinsed and drained)
- 1/2 cup cherry tomatoes, halved
- 1/2 cucumber, diced
- 1/4 cup red onion, finely chopped
- 1/4 cup chopped fresh parsley
- 2 tbsp olive oil
- 1 tbsp lemon juice
- Salt and pepper to taste

Directions:

1. **Prepare Vegetables:** Dice the cucumber, halve the cherry tomatoes, and chop the red onion and parsley.
2. **Combine Ingredients:** In a large bowl, mix the cooked quinoa, chickpeas, cherry tomatoes, cucumber, red onion, and parsley.
3. **Make Dressing:** In a small bowl, whisk together olive oil, lemon juice, salt, and pepper.
4. **Toss Salad:** Pour the dressing over the quinoa mixture and toss to combine.
5. **Serve:** Chill in the refrigerator for at least 30 minutes before serving.

Cooking and Prep Time:

- **Prep Time:** 15 minutes
- **Cooking Time:** None (if quinoa is pre-cooked)
- **Total Time:** 15 minutes (plus optional chilling time)

Servings: 2

Nutritional Information (per serving, approximate):

- Calories: 320
- Protein: 10g
- Carbohydrates: 40g
- Fiber: 8g
- Fat: 15g
- Saturated Fat: 2g
- Sodium: 300mg

2. Chicken and Vegetable Stir-Fry

Ingredients:

- 1 tbsp olive oil
- 1 cup boneless, skinless chicken breast, thinly sliced
- 1 cup broccoli florets
- 1/2 bell pepper, sliced
- 1/2 cup snap peas
- 2 tbsp low-sodium soy sauce
- 1 tbsp hoisin sauce (optional)
- 1 clove garlic, minced
- 1/2 tsp grated ginger
- 1 cup cooked brown rice

Directions:

1. **Prepare Vegetables:** Slice the bell pepper and trim the snap peas. Mince the garlic and grate the ginger.

2. **Cook Chicken:** Heat olive oil in a large skillet or wok over medium-high heat. Add sliced chicken and cook until no longer pink, about 5-7 minutes.
3. **Add Vegetables:** Add garlic, ginger, broccoli, bell pepper, and snap peas to the skillet. Stir-fry for 4-5 minutes until vegetables are tender-crisp.
4. **Add Sauces:** Stir in soy sauce and hoisin sauce (if using). Cook for another 2 minutes.
5. **Serve:** Serve the stir-fry over cooked brown rice.

Cooking and Prep Time:

- **Prep Time:** 10 minutes
- **Cooking Time:** 15 minutes
- **Total Time:** 25 minutes

Servings: 2

Nutritional Information (per serving, approximate):

- Calories: 400
- Protein: 30g
- Carbohydrates: 45g
- Fiber: 6g
- Fat: 10g
- Saturated Fat: 1.5g
- Sodium: 650mg

3. Lentil Soup with Spinach

Ingredients:

- 1 tbsp olive oil
- 1 onion, chopped
- 2 carrots, diced
- 2 celery stalks, diced

- 2 cloves garlic, minced
- 1 cup dried green or brown lentils, rinsed
- 4 cups vegetable broth
- 1 can diced tomatoes (14.5 oz)
- 2 cups fresh spinach
- 1 tsp dried thyme
- Salt and pepper to taste

Directions:

1. **Sauté Vegetables:** Heat olive oil in a large pot over medium heat. Add onion, carrots, and celery. Sauté until vegetables are softened, about 5 minutes.
2. **Add Garlic:** Stir in garlic and cook for an additional 1 minute.
3. **Cook Lentils:** Add lentils, vegetable broth, diced tomatoes, and dried thyme to the pot. Bring to a boil, then reduce heat and simmer for 25-30 minutes, or until lentils are tender.
4. **Add Spinach:** Stir in fresh spinach and cook for an additional 2-3 minutes until wilted.
5. **Season:** Season with salt and pepper to taste.

Cooking and Prep Time:

- **Prep Time:** 15 minutes
- **Cooking Time:** 30 minutes
- **Total Time:** 45 minutes

Servings: 4

Nutritional Information (per serving, approximate):

- Calories: 210
- Protein: 12g
- Carbohydrates: 35g

- Fiber: 10g
- Fat: 4g
- Saturated Fat: 1g
- Sodium: 400mg

5.3 Dinner Ideas

1. Baked Salmon with Asparagus and Quinoa

Ingredients:

- 2 salmon fillets (about 6 oz each)
- 1 bunch asparagus, trimmed
- 1 tbsp olive oil
- 1 lemon, sliced
- 1 tsp dried dill or fresh dill (optional)
- 1 cup cooked quinoa
- Salt and pepper to taste

Directions:

1. **Preheat Oven:** Preheat your oven to 400°F (200°C).
2. **Prepare Salmon:** Place salmon fillets on a baking sheet lined with parchment paper. Drizzle with olive oil, season with salt, pepper, and dill (if using). Top with lemon slices.
3. **Prepare Asparagus:** Toss asparagus with a little olive oil, salt, and pepper. Arrange around the salmon on the baking sheet.
4. **Bake:** Bake for 15-20 minutes, or until the salmon is cooked through and flakes easily with a fork, and asparagus is tender.
5. **Serve:** Serve the salmon and asparagus over a bed of cooked quinoa.

Cooking and Prep Time:

- **Prep Time:** 10 minutes
- **Cooking Time:** 20 minutes
- **Total Time:** 30 minutes

Servings: 2

Nutritional Information (per serving, approximate):

- Calories: 450
- Protein: 35g
- Carbohydrates: 35g
- Fiber: 6g
- Fat: 20g
- Saturated Fat: 3g
- Sodium: 150mg

2. Turkey and Vegetable Stuffed Bell Peppers

Ingredients:

- 4 large bell peppers (any color)
- 1 lb ground turkey
- 1 cup cooked brown rice
- 1 cup diced tomatoes (canned or fresh)
- 1/2 cup chopped onion
- 1/2 cup shredded cheese (optional, e.g., cheddar or mozzarella)
- 1 tsp dried oregano
- 1 tsp garlic powder
- Salt and pepper to taste

Directions:

1. **Preheat Oven:** Preheat your oven to 375°F (190°C).
2. **Prepare Peppers:** Cut the tops off the bell peppers and remove seeds and membranes. Set aside.

3. **Cook Filling:** In a skillet over medium heat, cook ground turkey with onion until browned and cooked through. Add diced tomatoes, cooked brown rice, oregano, garlic powder, salt, and pepper. Stir to combine and cook for 5 minutes.
4. **Stuff Peppers:** Spoon the turkey mixture into each bell pepper. Place stuffed peppers in a baking dish.
5. **Add Cheese:** Sprinkle shredded cheese on top of each pepper if using.
6. **Bake:** Bake for 25-30 minutes, or until peppers are tender and filling is heated through.

Cooking and Prep Time:

- **Prep Time:** 15 minutes
- **Cooking Time:** 30 minutes
- **Total Time:** 45 minutes

Servings: 4

Nutritional Information (per serving, approximate):

- Calories: 350
- Protein: 30g
- Carbohydrates: 35g
- Fiber: 7g
- Fat: 12g
- Saturated Fat: 5g
- Sodium: 300mg

3. Chicken and Sweet Potato Skillet

Ingredients:

- 2 boneless, skinless chicken breasts (about 6 oz each)

- 2 medium sweet potatoes, peeled and diced
- 1 tbsp olive oil
- 1/2 cup diced onion
- 2 cloves garlic, minced
- 1 tsp paprika
- 1/2 tsp ground cumin
- 1/2 tsp dried thyme
- Salt and pepper to taste
- 1 cup baby spinach (optional)

Directions:

1. **Cook Sweet Potatoes:** Heat olive oil in a large skillet over medium heat. Add diced sweet potatoes and cook, stirring occasionally, for about 10 minutes, or until they begin to soften.
2. **Add Onion and Garlic:** Stir in diced onion and garlic. Cook for another 2-3 minutes.
3. **Cook Chicken:** Season chicken breasts with paprika, cumin, thyme, salt, and pepper. Place chicken in the skillet with sweet potatoes. Cook for about 7-8 minutes on each side, or until chicken is cooked through and sweet potatoes are tender.
4. **Add Spinach (Optional):** Stir in baby spinach if using, and cook for an additional 1-2 minutes until wilted.
5. **Serve:** Slice the chicken and serve with the sweet potato mixture.

Cooking and Prep Time:

- **Prep Time:** 10 minutes
- **Cooking Time:** 20 minutes
- **Total Time:** 30 minutes

Servings: 2

Nutritional Information (per serving, approximate):

- Calories: 400
- Protein: 35g
- Carbohydrates: 35g
- Fiber: 6g
- Fat: 12g
- Saturated Fat: 2g
- Sodium: 200mg

5.4 Snacks

1. Hummus and Veggie Sticks

Ingredients:

- 1 cup store-bought or homemade hummus
- 1 large carrot, cut into sticks
- 1 large cucumber, cut into sticks
- 1 red bell pepper, cut into sticks
- 1 cup cherry tomatoes

Directions:

1. **Prepare Vegetables:** Wash and cut the carrot, cucumber, and red bell pepper into sticks.
2. **Serve:** Arrange the vegetable sticks and cherry tomatoes on a plate. Serve with a cup of hummus for dipping.

Cooking and Prep Time:

- **Prep Time:** 10 minutes
- **Cooking Time:** None
- **Total Time:** 10 minutes

Servings: 2

Nutritional Information (per serving, approximate):

- Calories: 180
- Protein: 6g
- Carbohydrates: 22g
- Fiber: 8g
- Fat: 8g

- Saturated Fat: 1g
- Sodium: 300mg

2. Greek Yogurt with Honey and Almonds

Ingredients:

- 1 cup plain Greek yogurt
- 1 tbsp honey
- 2 tbsp sliced almonds

Directions:

1. **Prepare Yogurt:** Scoop the Greek yogurt into a bowl.
2. **Add Toppings:** Drizzle the honey over the yogurt and sprinkle with sliced almonds.
3. **Serve:** Serve immediately or refrigerate until ready to eat.

Cooking and Prep Time:

- **Prep Time:** 5 minutes
- **Cooking Time:** None
- **Total Time:** 5 minutes

Servings: 1

Nutritional Information (per serving, approximate):

- Calories: 240
- Protein: 18g
- Carbohydrates: 22g
- Fiber: 2g
- Fat: 9g

- Saturated Fat: 1g
- Sodium: 70mg

3. Apple Slices with Peanut Butter

Ingredients:

- 1 large apple (any variety), sliced
- 2 tbsp natural peanut butter

Directions:

1. **Prepare Apple:** Wash and slice the apple into wedges.
2. **Serve:** Arrange the apple slices on a plate and serve with peanut butter for dipping.

Cooking and Prep Time:

- **Prep Time:** 5 minutes
- **Cooking Time:** None
- **Total Time:** 5 minutes

Servings: 1

Nutritional Information (per serving, approximate):

- Calories: 210
- Protein: 4g
- Carbohydrates: 30g
- Fiber: 5g
- Fat: 9g
- Saturated Fat: 1.5g
- Sodium: 2mg

5.5 Desserts

1. Chia Seed Pudding with Berries

Ingredients:

- 1/4 cup chia seeds
- 1 cup unsweetened almond milk (or any milk of choice)
- 1 tbsp honey or maple syrup
- 1/2 tsp vanilla extract
- 1/2 cup mixed berries (strawberries, blueberries, raspberries)

Directions:

1. **Combine Ingredients:** In a bowl or jar, mix chia seeds, almond milk, honey (or maple syrup), and vanilla extract.
2. **Refrigerate:** Stir well and let sit for 5 minutes. Stir again to prevent clumping. Cover and refrigerate for at least 4 hours, or overnight.
3. **Serve:** When ready to serve, top with mixed berries.

Cooking and Prep Time:

- **Prep Time:** 10 minutes
- **Refrigeration Time:** 4 hours (minimum)
- **Total Time:** 4 hours 10 minutes

Servings: 2

Nutritional Information (per serving, approximate):

- Calories: 200
- Protein: 5g
- Carbohydrates: 28g

- Fiber: 12g
- Fat: 8g
- Saturated Fat: 1g
- Sodium: 80mg

2. Baked Apple with Cinnamon and Walnuts

Ingredients:

- 2 large apples (any variety)
- 2 tsp cinnamon
- 2 tbsp chopped walnuts
- 2 tsp honey or maple syrup

Directions:

1. **Preheat Oven:** Preheat your oven to 350°F (175°C).
2. **Prepare Apples:** Core the apples and place them in a baking dish. Sprinkle with cinnamon and fill the centers with chopped walnuts. Drizzle with honey or maple syrup.
3. **Bake:** Bake for 25-30 minutes, or until the apples are tender.
4. **Serve:** Let cool slightly before serving.

Cooking and Prep Time:

- **Prep Time:** 10 minutes
- **Cooking Time:** 25-30 minutes
- **Total Time:** 35-40 minutes

Servings: 2

Nutritional Information (per serving, approximate):

- Calories: 180
- Protein: 2g
- Carbohydrates: 36g
- Fiber: 6g
- Fat: 5g
- Saturated Fat: 0.5g
- Sodium: 0mg

3. Greek Yogurt Parfait with Granola and Fruit

Ingredients:

- 1 cup plain Greek yogurt
- 1/2 cup granola (choose a low-sugar variety)
- 1/2 cup mixed fresh fruit (e.g., berries, kiwi, banana)
- 1 tsp honey or maple syrup (optional)

Directions:

1. **Layer Ingredients:** In a glass or bowl, layer half of the Greek yogurt, followed by half of the granola and fruit. Repeat with the remaining yogurt, granola, and fruit.
2. **Top with Sweetener (Optional):** Drizzle with honey or maple syrup if desired.
3. **Serve:** Serve immediately.

Cooking and Prep Time:

- **Prep Time:** 5 minutes
- **Cooking Time:** None
- **Total Time:** 5 minutes

Servings: 1

Nutritional Information (per serving, approximate):

- Calories: 300
- Protein: 16g
- Carbohydrates: 45g
- Fiber: 6g
- Fat: 9g
- Saturated Fat: 1g
- Sodium: 100mg

5.5 Sample Weekly Meal Plan

Day 1

Breakfast: Greek Yogurt with Honey and Almonds

Snack: Apple Slices with Peanut Butter

Lunch: Quinoa Salad with Chickpeas and Vegetables

Snack: Hummus and Veggie Sticks

Dinner: Baked Salmon with Asparagus and Quinoa

Dessert: Chia Seed Pudding with Berries

Day 2

Breakfast: Chia Seed Pudding with Berries

Snack: Hummus and Veggie Sticks

Lunch: Chicken and Vegetable Stir-Fry

Snack: Greek Yogurt with Honey and Almonds

Dinner: Turkey and Vegetable Stuffed Bell Peppers

Dessert: Baked Apple with Cinnamon and Walnuts

Day 3

Breakfast: Greek Yogurt Parfait with Granola and Fruit

Snack: Apple Slices with Peanut Butter

Lunch: Lentil Soup with Spinach

Snack: Greek Yogurt with Honey and Almonds

Dinner: Chicken and Sweet Potato Skillet

Dessert: Greek Yogurt Parfait with Granola and Fruit

Day 4

Breakfast: Greek Yogurt with Honey and Almonds

Snack: Hummus and Veggie Sticks

Lunch: Quinoa Salad with Chickpeas and Vegetables

Snack: Apple Slices with Peanut Butter

Dinner: Baked Salmon with Asparagus and Quinoa

Dessert: Chia Seed Pudding with Berries

Day 5

Breakfast: Chia Seed Pudding with Berries

Snack: Greek Yogurt with Honey and Almonds

Lunch: Chicken and Vegetable Stir-Fry

Snack: Hummus and Veggie Sticks

Dinner: Turkey and Vegetable Stuffed Bell Peppers

Dessert: Baked Apple with Cinnamon and Walnuts

Day 6

Breakfast: Greek Yogurt Parfait with Granola and Fruit

Snack: Apple Slices with Peanut Butter

Lunch: Lentil Soup with Spinach

Snack: Greek Yogurt with Honey and Almonds

Dinner: Chicken and Sweet Potato Skillet

Dessert: Greek Yogurt Parfait with Granola and Fruit

Day 7

Breakfast: Greek Yogurt with Honey and Almonds

Snack: Hummus and Veggie Sticks

Lunch: Quinoa Salad with Chickpeas and Vegetables

Snack: Apple Slices with Peanut Butter

Dinner: Baked Salmon with Asparagus and Quinoa

Dessert: Chia Seed Pudding with Berries

Chapter 6: Glycemic Index and Chronic Conditions

6.1 Diabetes Management

Managing diabetes involves careful monitoring of blood glucose levels, and the Glycemic Index (GI) can play a crucial role in this process. The GI measures how quickly carbohydrates in foods raise blood glucose levels. Food sources with a high GI cause a fast spike in glucose, while those with a low GI bring about a more slow, more steady increment.

Benefits of Using the GI for Diabetes Management:

1. **Improved Blood Sugar Control:** By choosing low-GI foods, individuals with diabetes can better manage their blood glucose levels, reducing the risk of hyperglycemia (high blood sugar) and hypoglycemia (low blood sugar).
2. **Enhanced Insulin Sensitivity:** Low-GI foods help improve insulin sensitivity, making it easier for the body to use insulin effectively.
3. **Reduced Risk of Complications:** Consistently managing blood glucose levels can help prevent long-term complications associated with diabetes, such as cardiovascular disease, nerve damage, and kidney problems.

Practical Tips for Using the GI:

- **Select Low-GI Foods:** Incorporate more whole grains, legumes, fruits, and non-starchy vegetables into your diet.
- **Balance Meals:** Combine carbohydrates with proteins and healthy fats to lower the overall GI of a meal and slow glucose absorption.
- **Monitor Portion Sizes:** Even low-GI foods can impact blood sugar if consumed in large quantities, so portion control is essential.
- **Consistency:** Aim for regular meal times and consistent carbohydrate intake throughout the day to maintain stable blood glucose levels.

By understanding and utilizing the Glycemic Index, individuals with diabetes can make informed dietary choices that support effective blood sugar management and overall health.

6.2 Heart Disease Prevention

Heart disease is a leading cause of morbidity and mortality, particularly among seniors. Managing diet through the Glycemic Index (GI) can play a significant role in heart disease prevention. The GI helps individuals select foods that not only support stable blood sugar levels but also contribute to overall heart health.

Benefits of Using the GI for Heart Disease Prevention:

1. **Improved Cholesterol Levels:** Low-GI foods tend to be high in fiber, particularly soluble fiber, which can help lower LDL (bad) cholesterol levels. This, in turn, reduces the risk of atherosclerosis, a condition where the arteries become clogged and can lead to heart attacks and strokes.
2. **Better Weight Management:** Keeping a solid weight is urgent for heart wellbeing. Low-GI foods help control appetite and reduce hunger, making it easier to manage weight effectively.
3. **Reduced Inflammation:** High-GI foods can cause spikes in blood sugar that may lead to increased inflammation, a risk factor for heart disease. By choosing low-GI options, individuals can help reduce systemic inflammation.

Practical Tips for Using the GI for Heart Disease Prevention:

- **Focus on Whole Foods:** Incorporate more whole grains, fruits, vegetables, legumes, and nuts into your diet. These foods are generally lower in GI and high in essential nutrients.
- **Healthy Fats:** Include sources of healthy fats such as avocados, olive oil, and fatty fish. These fats are beneficial for heart health and can help lower the overall GI of meals.
- **Limit Processed Foods:** Minimize consumption of processed and refined foods, such as white bread, pastries, and sugary snacks, which typically have a high GI and contribute to heart disease risk.

- **Balance Carbohydrate Intake:** Pair carbohydrates with proteins and healthy fats to lower the glycemic impact of meals and promote more stable blood sugar levels.

By understanding and incorporating the principles of the Glycemic Index into their diet, seniors can take proactive steps towards preventing heart disease. This approach not only helps manage blood sugar but also supports overall cardiovascular health, contributing to a longer and healthier life.

6.3 Managing Weight

Maintaining a healthy weight is essential for overall well-being, especially for seniors. The Glycemic Index (GI) can be a useful tool in managing weight effectively by helping individuals choose foods that promote satiety and stabilize blood sugar levels.

Benefits of Using the GI for Weight Management:

1. **Enhanced Satiety:** Low-GI foods are digested and absorbed more slowly, leading to prolonged feelings of fullness. This diminishes in general calorie admission by controlling hunger and forestalling gorging.
2. **Stable Blood Sugar Levels:** High-GI foods cause rapid spikes and subsequent drops in blood sugar, which can trigger hunger and cravings. Low-GI foods help maintain stable blood sugar levels, reducing the likelihood of these fluctuations and aiding in appetite control.
3. **Reduced Fat Storage:** Frequent spikes in blood sugar can lead to increased insulin production, which promotes fat storage. By choosing low-GI foods, seniors can help minimize insulin spikes and reduce the tendency to store fat.

Practical Tips for Using the GI for Weight Management:

- **Incorporate Fiber-Rich Foods:** High-fiber foods such as whole grains, legumes, fruits, and vegetables typically have a low GI and are excellent for promoting satiety and digestion.
- **Combine Macronutrients:** Pair carbohydrates with proteins and healthy fats to slow down the absorption of sugars, which helps keep blood sugar levels stable and prolongs satiety.
- **Choose Whole Foods Over Processed Foods:** Processed foods often have a high GI and are less filling than whole foods. Opt for minimally processed options to improve satiety and nutrient intake.

- **Mind Portion Sizes:** Even low-GI foods can contribute to weight gain if consumed in excessive amounts. Be aware of part sizes to successfully oversee calorie consumption.
- **Stay Hydrated:** Sometimes, thirst is mistaken for hunger. Drinking plenty of water can help manage appetite and support overall health.

By integrating the principles of the Glycemic Index into their dietary habits, seniors can manage their weight more effectively, promoting better health and a higher quality of life. This approach not only aids in weight control but also contributes to overall metabolic health and well-being.

6.4 Digestive Health

Maintaining good digestive health is crucial for overall well-being, particularly for seniors. The Glycemic Index (GI) can play a significant role in supporting digestive health by guiding food choices that promote efficient digestion and gut health.

Benefits of Using the GI for Digestive Health:

1. **Improved Digestive Regularity:** Low-GI foods are often rich in dietary fiber, which is essential for maintaining regular bowel movements and preventing constipation.
2. **Enhanced Gut Flora:** Many low-GI foods, such as fruits, vegetables, legumes, and whole grains, contain prebiotics that support the growth of beneficial gut bacteria. A healthy gut microbiome is vital for efficient digestion and nutrient absorption.
3. **Reduced Digestive Discomfort:** High-GI foods can lead to rapid spikes in blood sugar, which may cause digestive discomfort and bloating. Low-GI foods help maintain a steadier digestive process, reducing the likelihood of these issues.

Practical Tips for Using the GI for Digestive Health:

- **Increase Fiber Intake:** Incorporate more high-fiber, low-GI foods into your diet, such as whole grains, legumes, fruits, and vegetables. Fiber aids in digestion and helps keep the digestive tract running smoothly.
- **Stay Hydrated:** Sufficient hydration is fundamental for appropriate processing. Drinking plenty of water helps fiber work more effectively and prevents constipation.
- **Chew Thoroughly:** Take time to chew food thoroughly, which aids in the digestive process and allows for better absorption of nutrients.

- **Avoid Highly Processed Foods:** Processed foods often have a high GI and can be low in fiber. Opt for whole, minimally processed foods to support digestive health.
- **Monitor Portion Sizes:** Eating large meals can overwhelm the digestive system. Smaller, more frequent meals can be easier on digestion and help maintain steady blood sugar levels.

Dietary Habits for Optimal Digestive Health:

- **Regular Meal Times:** Consistent meal times help regulate digestion and improve overall digestive health.
- **Mindful Eating:** Eat slowly and mindfully to support the digestive process and prevent overeating.
- **Incorporate Probiotics:** Foods like yogurt, kefir, and fermented vegetables provide beneficial probiotics that promote a healthy gut.

By focusing on low-GI foods and incorporating these dietary habits, seniors can enhance their digestive health, leading to better nutrient absorption, improved regularity, and overall well-being. A healthy digestive system contributes significantly to overall health, making it an important aspect of dietary management for seniors.

Chapter 7: Conclusion

The **Glycemic Index Food Guide Chart for Seniors 2024** provides a comprehensive resource for understanding how food choices impact blood sugar levels and overall health. As we age, maintaining a balanced diet becomes increasingly important, and the Glycemic Index (GI) is a valuable tool in achieving this balance.

Through the chapters of this guide, we have explored the fundamental concepts of the GI, how it is measured, and the differences between the Glycemic Index and Glycemic Load. We have delved into the health benefits of low-GI foods, including their roles in managing diabetes, supporting heart health, aiding in weight management, and promoting digestive health.

Understanding the factors that influence the GI of foods, such as types of carbohydrates, fiber content, ripeness, processing, cooking methods, and food combinations, empowers seniors to make informed dietary choices. This guide has provided practical tips for incorporating low-GI options into daily meals, with specific sections dedicated to various food categories, from fruits and vegetables to grains, dairy products, protein sources, and snacks.

The sample meal plans and recipes offer a practical framework for integrating low-GI foods into a balanced diet. These plans are designed to be both nutritious and delicious, ensuring that seniors can enjoy their meals while reaping the health benefits of low-GI eating.

By following the guidelines and suggestions in this book, seniors can better manage their blood sugar levels, reduce the risk of chronic diseases, maintain a healthy weight, and support overall well-being. The Glycemic Index is not just a tool for managing specific health conditions; it is a holistic approach to healthier living.

As we conclude this guide, we encourage you to take the knowledge and insights gained here and apply them to your daily life. Embrace the variety of low-GI foods, experiment with new recipes, and enjoy the journey towards a healthier, more vibrant you. Remember, the choices you make today can significantly impact your health and quality of life in the years to come.

Thank you for using the **Glycemic Index Food Guide Chart for Seniors 2024**. We hope it serves as a valuable companion on your path to better health and well-being.